Doing a Literature Review in Health and Social Care
A practical guide

Doing a
Literature Review in
Health and
Social Care

A practical guide

Third edition

Helen Aveyard

 Open University Press

Open University Press
McGraw-Hill Education
McGraw-Hill House
Shoppenhangers Road
Maidenhead
Berkshire
England
SL6 2QL

email: enquiries@openup.co.uk
world wide web: www.openup.co.uk

and Two Penn Plaza, New York, NY 10121–2289, USA

First published 2007
First published in the second edition 2010
First published in this third edition 2014

A catalogue record of this book is available from the British Library

ISBN-13: 978-0-33-526307-3 (pb)
ISBN-10: 0-33-526307-0 (pb)
eISBN: 978-0-33-526308-0

Library of Congress Cataloging-in-Publication Data
CIP data applied for

Typesetting and e-book compilations by
RefineCatch Limited, Bungay, Suffolk

Printed and bound by Bell and Bain Ltd, Glasgow

MIX
Paper from
responsible sources
FSC® C007785

Praise for this book

"This deceptively small book provides a comprehensive, user-friendly, step-by-step guide to the development of a literature review. Key strengths are the clarity of expression and the logical flow of information. Chapters match the stages of a literature review, from start to finish. Useful examples and key questions will help to keep the reader on track. With this book as your guide, developing a literature review need not be a daunting or overwhelming task."

Dr Merryl E Harvey, Senior Academic, Faculty of Health,
Birmingham City University, UK

Amazon reviews for the 2nd edition

"This really helped me complete my dissertation. Well set out, easy to understand and for literature review beginners a very good place to start."

"This book has really helped me understand what a literature review is, and gives great insight into what is expected from your literature review."

"Buy this book: it's a god send!"

Contents

Foreword

Some have made an art and a science and, indeed, a living out of literature reviewing – or their version of it. Something that was once relatively simple, and was done with little semblance of rigour, has been elevated from a literary technique to a full-fledged research method. While the development in reviewing is largely to be welcomed, I have some reservations.

I use the term 'reviewing' deliberately, without qualification or prefix, since there is a range of ways of conducting reviews and these all aim to do the same thing and all stem from the same desire. They have been developed for the same purpose. People want to know what is 'out there', for many reasons, and there are several ways to do this; I also believe that different types of literature review suit different purposes. The 'art' lies in realizing what is similar across the range of methods, and their common purpose; the 'science' lies in selecting the right methods and conducting your review to the highest standards that are both necessary and possible.

The problem is that some of the cognoscenti in the world of reviewing have also established themselves at the top of a hierarchy and appear only to have an interest in either kicking over the ladder for those trying to learn, or for making the art and science of reviewing so elusive that few can follow.

What faces, for example, the early stage postgraduate research student setting out to explore the literature – doing their 'literature review' – is an array of methods ranging from narrative review to meta-analysis and not a single method called 'literature review' in sight. They will have come across the term 'systematic review' or been advised that they have to do a systematic review as part of their doctoral programme. Imagine the confusion of the poor student who searches the Internet for 'systematic review' and finds only information on meta-analysis with its bubble plots and confidence intervals. This dismay is often confounded by colleagues who tell them that the term 'systematic review' is reserved for meta-analysis and that everything else is just a plain, and by implication poor, literature review. I have even heard an external examiner tell a PhD student that what they had done was not a systematic review when it clearly was. So what?

The advent of information technology, the widespread use of personal computers and the development of apps for smart phones and tablets mean that literature reviewing is literally at the fingertips of almost anyone. This is a good thing but people cannot necessarily be let loose with the method. Therefore, literature reviewing is very important, and it is far too important to be left only to the experts. Like knowing the basic tenets of an experiment or how a cohort study and a panel study differ, knowing how to review the literature is essential for all health and social care practitioners, whether in clinical practice or in research.

Enter the third edition of Helen Aveyard's *Doing a Literature Review in Health and Social Care: A Practical Guide*. This book is the perfect antidote to those who have been inflicted by confusion having tried to learn what a literature review is from a local expert, a book on research methods or the Internet. The distinction between a regular systematic review and a meta-analysis is made early and the value of the systematic review without meta-analysis is also stated. This will be a great relief to many. Otherwise, the budding literature reviewer – and many with experience – will find all that they need in this book. There are practical examples of why reviews are necessary and where they have been used, as well as excellent and simple guidance on how to do different types of reviews. Three editions of this book attest to its utility. In this fast-moving area of research, and with the primacy of systematic reviews in this age of evidence-based practice, I envisage further editions.

Roger Watson PhD RN FRCN FAAN
Professor of Nursing
Editor-in-Chief, *Journal of Advanced Nursing*
University of Hull, Hull, UK

Acknowledgements

I would like to thank the following individuals for their help during the writing of this book.

Jill Gregory for proof reading the manuscript

Paul, Benedict and Edward Aveyard for being there

Introduction

If you are reading this book, you are probably about to embark on a project or dissertation in which you will undertake a review of the literature. In some cases, your literature review will be a preliminary investigation prior to undertaking a larger research project. In other cases, your literature review will form the entire project in which the literature is reviewed in order to answer a particular question. In this case, the literature review may be the dissertation component for your undergraduate or postgraduate degree in nursing, health or social care. Whichever the requirement of your literature review, this book will guide you through the process of developing a literature review question, searching, appraising and analysing the literature so that you can develop a comprehensive and systematic approach to your review.

A literature review is the comprehensive study and interpretation of literature that addresses a specific topic. If your literature review is a preliminary review prior to a larger study, the purpose of the review will be to provide a critical account of the literature in a particular area in order to demonstrate why a new research study is required. The aim of the review will be to identify and critique the existing literature on the topic of enquiry, in order to demonstrate a gap in the existing research base and to *justify* your proposed plan of research. In addition, exploration of existing research and the methods used to investigate the area will add to your understanding of the topic as a whole.

If the entire focus of your project is a literature review, you will seek to *answer* a specific question in your review. In this case, the purpose of the review will be to provide new insights into a research question by reviewing existing literature rather than provide a justification for a new study, although you may well conclude that there is insufficient literature to answer your question and hence a new study is recommended.

For both approaches to the literature review, it is important that you develop and maintain a comprehensive approach to undertaking your review. Sometimes you will hear the term 'systematic review' – this refers to a review that is undertaken in great detail, which we will discuss later on in this book. A truly 'systematic' review is generally considered to be beyond the remit of most undergraduate and even postgraduate projects. However, the principles of a systematic review – that it be carried out in a comprehensive and logical manner – are those that can and should be adhered to by anyone undertaking a literature review.

More and more students are undertaking a literature review as part of their undergraduate or postgraduate degree for the following reasons. First, research ethics committees and local research governance procedures are increasingly rigorous in their review of student projects, and the time taken to prepare a submission for each committee can take many months. This is often a prohibitive factor for students aiming to undertake studies involving primary data collection. For pragmatic reasons, many students within nursing, midwifery, social work, occupational therapy and physiotherapy undertake literature-based dissertations instead.

Second, literature reviews are becoming ever more important in health and social care. The growing importance of evidence-based practice (EBP) within health and social care today has led to literature reviews becoming more relevant to current practice. The emphasis on 'knowledge summaries', of which literature reviews are often a central component, is an example of this. In a literature review, all the available evidence on any given topic is retrieved and reviewed so that an overall picture of what is known about the topic is achieved. The value of one individual piece of research is greater if it is seen in the context of other literature on the same topic. Thus the literature review is regarded as increasingly important in health and social care and the method for undertaking a literature review has become an important research methodology in its own right.

How this book is presented

In this book, the steps involved in doing your literature review are outlined and an approach to undertaking a literature review using a systematic approach is described. This approach is suitable for everyone who is new to, or has little experience of, this process and reflects the approach undertaken by experts. While the focus of this book is the literature review that forms the entire project and seeks to answer a specific question, rather than the review which forms the preliminary stages of a larger research project, the principles of undertaking both types of review are similar; it is the aims and conclusions of the reviews that are different.

Undertaking a literature review is complex and has defined theoretical underpinnings about which you need to be aware if you are undertaking a review of your own. Some of the arguments are complex and will be addressed and simplified in this book. Yet in general terms, all literature reviews undertaken for an undergraduate or postgraduate degree should be 'systematic' – even if not in the detail of a full systematic review – and you will be given greater credit the more detailed your review is. This book will equip you with the knowledge and skills to do this successfully.

This book also promotes a systematic approach to the literature review process for the novice researcher. It summarizes the current debate surrounding the process of undertaking a literature review and then gives a clear guide to searching for, critiquing and finally bringing together the literature to form a review. This book is an ideal resource for undergraduate students who are undertaking a dissertation. It is also intended as an introductory text for those studying at postgraduate level or who are new to the process of reviewing the literature. Furthermore, it is an ideal text for practitioners who are returning to study or who are updating their skills in continuing professional development. This book will give you a step-by-step guide to undertaking a systematic approach to your literature review.

What's in the third edition?

The latest ideas and developments in searching for and appraising literature are incorporated in this new edition. In particular, there is a focus on the way in which you can incorporate critical appraisal into a literature review without losing sight of the results of the study and how you can combine the results of your review in an easy to follow thematic analysis. As in the first and second editions, the book is written in an accessible, student-friendly way. Furthermore, many more examples are included of commonly occurring real-life scenarios encountered by students in a variety of health and social care disciplines. The following is a summary of chapter contents:

- **Chapter 1: Why do a literature review in health and social care?** To begin, you are introduced to the importance of literature reviews, the different types of literature review that exist and what makes a literature review different from other kinds of research and academic writing.

- **Chapter 2: How do I develop a question for my literature review?** In this chapter, the process of developing a question for your review is explored, with an emphasis that good questions often arise from your practice area. This chapter has been updated to emphasize the importance of setting a question at the very start of your project. The research question articulates the purpose of the review and ensures that the review has a specific focus rather than a general discussion of a particular topic. A step-by-step guide to developing your question is given with reference to different formulas to guide your question development and with specific reference to your professional practice.
- **Chapter 3: Which literature will be relevant to my literature review?** In this chapter, the importance of identifying which literature is relevant to your review is discussed. Emphasis is put on recognizing the type of literature that is needed to address different literature review questions, which is usually, but not always, research. This chapter has been updated to provide a clear guide to the types of literature you are likely to come across.
- **Chapter 4: How do I search for literature?** In this chapter, the process of undertaking a thorough and systematic search is discussed. The importance of stating clear inclusion and exclusion criteria for the literature you seek is emphasized. These inclusion and exclusion criteria will reflect the decisions about the literature you include as discussed in Chapter 3.
- **Chapter 5: How do I critically appraise the literature?** In this chapter, the process of critical appraisal of the literature you identify is discussed together with discussion about the pros and cons of omitting literature from your review due to quality indicators. This chapter has been updated to provide a wide range of critical appraisal tools.
- **Chapter 6: How do I analyse my findings?** Bringing together the results of your review can be a complex and daunting process. This chapter contains an updated and simplified approach to combining literature in a review. The different methods of comparing and contrasting the literature are discussed. A method suitable for those new to the literature review process is outlined.
- **Chapter 7: How do I discuss my findings and make recommendations?** In this chapter, the writing of appropriate conclusions and recommendations is discussed. It is essential that conclusions and recommendations can be seen to have arisen directly from the results of your literature review, rather than from any preconceived ideas that you may have had.
- **Chapter 8: Frequently asked questions.** Here you will find answers to some of the most commonly asked questions that arise when

students are undertaking a literature review, including how to structure your review, the importance of appropriate referencing and academic rigour throughout the process of writing a literature review.

At the end of the book, after Chapter 8, you will find a Glossary of all the key terms you might need. As you read through the book, you will see these key terms highlighted in the text the first time they are used to indicate that they are included in the Glossary. Use this Glossary as you read through or for quick reference once you have finished.

1

Why do a literature review in health and social care?

What is a literature review?

Let's begin by defining what a literature review is. In short, a literature review is the comprehensive study and interpretation of literature that relates to a particular topic. When you undertake a literature review, you identify a **research question** and then seek to answer this question by searching for and **analysing** relevant literature using a systematic approach. This is the case whether your literature review is a pre-requirement to a larger project or is a study in its own right. A thorough search and analysis of the literature leads you to new insights that are only possible when all the literature is reviewed together and each piece of relevant information is seen in the context of other information. If you think of one piece of literature as one part of a jigsaw, then you can see how a review of the literature is like the whole completed jigsaw. This is why a literature review is so useful.

What types of literature review are there?

As the demand for literature reviews has increased, so has the number of different approaches to undertaking a literature review. Arksey and O'Malley (2005) refer to the different terms that might be used to refer to a literature review, including: systematic review, rapid review, critical review, narrative review, structured review, scoping studies review.

A simplified approach is to consider what we mean by a literature review and then to look at the different reviews you come across in the light of this, rather than to consider the terminology used to describe the review. Some very detailed literature reviews are referred to as **systematic reviews.** These are described later in this chapter and refer to a very high quality literature review, generally undertaken by a team of researchers who aim to identify *all* the available evidence on a topic, undertake a thorough appraisal of the quality of the evidence and often include a re-analysis of results of the studies – sometimes referred to as a **meta-analysis** or **meta-synthesis**. This very detailed approach is beyond the scope and remit of an undergraduate and (often) postgraduate study.

If it is not possible to undertake a full systematic review, due to a lack of time and other resources, it is always possible for researchers to strive for a systematic approach to their review. In Aveyard and Sharp (2013) we discuss the *good quality literature review*, which is one that attempts to incorporate a systematic approach to literature searching, appraisal and re-analysis, even though the final review might fall short of a full and detailed systematic approach. One of the ways you can assess the quality of a literature review is to consider the way it has been done. A good quality literature review will be undertaken in a comprehensive way but not in the detail of a systematic review and probably without a team of researchers. It will contain a description of how the literature was searched and how the quality of the literature was evaluated. It is usually possible to undertake a good quality literature review at undergraduate or postgraduate level. If you are intending to undertake a literature review as a component of your undergraduate or postgraduate degree, this is what you are likely to be aiming for.

The literature review as a research method

It is important to remember that a good quality literature review is a piece of research in its own right. As such, a literature review will follow the stages of the research process, incorporating a defined research question which is then answered using a pre-defined methodology involving searching for relevant literature, appraising and evaluating the literature, and combining the results. New insights are developed which address the research question, or indicate gaps in the current knowledge base, which point to the need for further study. It is important to document the stages in the research process of a literature review as for any other piece of research.

Literature reviews should usually adhere to the following structure:

- a literature review question (or research question) set in context within an introductory chapter
- a methods section incorporating your search strategy, method of appraisal and analysis of the literature
- presentation of your results/themes incorporating critical appraisal of the studies included
- discussion of your results and recommendations for practice.

You would expect to find the above process in all good quality literature reviews and systematic reviews. Sadly, it is still all too common to come across 'literature reviews' in many popular health and social care journals which do not adhere to this standard. Such 'reviews' often reference other research studies but fail to give a method by which the review was completed, and therefore the reader cannot tell if a comprehensive range of relevant literature was accessed and how this was evaluated and the review written up. If you come across a review that refers to lots of research but does not demonstrate a clear process as to how the review was undertaken, then this is not a systematic review or a good quality literature review and you should regard the results with caution. You should certainly not see this as a model upon which to base your undergraduate or postgraduate study!

Why are literature reviews important?

Literature reviews are important because they seek to summarize the literature that is available on any one topic. They make sense of a body of research and present an analysis of the available literature so that the reader does not have to access each individual research report included in the review. This is important because there is an increasing amount of literature available to all health and social care professionals, who cannot be expected to read and assimilate all the information on any one topic. Everyone who works within health and social care has a professional duty to be up to date with recent developments and research that informs their practice, otherwise they risk providing out of date care. Yet, it is virtually impossible for any one practitioner to assimilate, process and decide how to implement all this information in their professional lives. This is why literature reviews, in which all the research about a particular topic is brought together, are so important. If a practitioner reads only one report on a topic, it is possible to get a misleading picture, because that report is only one of many.

Literature reviews provide an overview of research in a specific area

---

One piece of evidence is only ever one piece of a larger jigsaw

Take, for example, the recent publicity surrounding information about smoking and smoking cessation. A recent Department of Health publicity campaign (DoH 2012) addresses the impact of smoking even a small number of cigarettes; the campaign states that smoking 15 cigarettes can lead to mutations that can lead to cancer. This claim is based on work undertaken by Pleasance et al. (2010) and The Wellcome Trust (2010). Contrast this with some of the results of the 'Million Women Study' (Pirie et al. 2013), which confirmed previous findings that the negative effects of smoking can be reduced by 97 per cent if an individual quits smoking at the age of 30 and by 90 per cent if he or she quits by the age of 40. At first glance, the message from these two pieces of information might seem to be contradictory – in one we are told that every 15 cigarettes is leading to harmful mutations and in the other we are told that the health risks of smoking up until the age of 30 or even 40 are, to a great extent, reversible.

Yet if we look at these two pieces of information in the context of others, we begin to see the bigger picture. Fifteen cigarettes *may* lead to mutations which *may* lead to cancer. And while the health risks associated with cancer are to some extent reversible, if an individual quits smoking by the age of 30, the risks are even less if you never smoke at all.

There are always pieces of literature that do not quite seem to fit together with the main body of research. Very occasionally, these are genuine 'red herrings' – take, for example, the Measles, Mumps and Rubella (MMR) vaccination controversy and the paper that initiated the scare about a possible link with the vaccination and autism and bowel disease (Wakefield et al. 1998), which was subsequently discredited. This paper can be regarded as a 'red herring'. It caused widespread public concern, which led to a reduction in uptake of the MMR vaccination, the effects of which are still ongoing at the time of writing (Kmietowicz 2012), including a large-scale measles outbreak in 2013 (Wise 2013). The paper was retracted due to concern about the **rigour** of the initial study and potential conflict of interests held by the authors of the paper. Furthermore, an extensive body of further research has failed to find any link as suggested by Wakefield and colleagues.

Another reason why a piece of literature might, at first glance, seem 'at odds' with the rest of the literature in a specific area, can be the way it is reported by the media; we are all familiar with the way in which information can be distorted and twisted to fit into a particular news story, and this illustrates why it is so important to track back to the original research rather than rely on media representation of a research report.

Literature reviews lessen the impact of individual pieces of research

Most frequently, however, different pieces of research and other evidence work together to build up a consistent picture of a particular area and one that you would not get by looking at one piece of information alone. This is why it is important to assess the value and contribution of any one article in the light of other articles that address the same topic in a literature review, rather than to make a conclusion from the findings of one paper that you read – for example, 'it's OK to quit at 30!' or 'every 15 cigarettes is irreversibly damaging me!' The findings of single research papers are not enough – or should not be enough – to influence practice. You can see how much more useful it is to see all the studies on a topic together in order to appreciate the whole picture. In this way, an academic judgement can be made about the contribution that all the information makes to our understanding of a particular area rather than a judgement made on one small piece of published information. This is why literature reviews are so important.

Analysis of many papers can lead to new discoveries

Literature reviews are important because new insights can be developed by reviewing all the research together, and these insights are not available without reviewing all of the research in a particular area. For example, Anderson *et al.* (2009) conducted a systematic review exploring the role of breast-feeding in the prevention of allergies in babies and young children. This was done by searching for all studies on the topic and then by comparing the findings of one study with the findings of others. As a result, a clearer understanding of the role of breast-feeding and allergies was developed which has influenced health advice given to new mothers.

Sometimes it is possible to compare studies in more detail, by combining the statistical data from many smaller studies and re-analysing the data as if it was one larger study. This enables researchers to see the full impact of the results of many studies combined together, which, read in isolation, may not appear that significant. This process of combining the statistical results of many studies, where it is appropriate to do so, is known as **meta-analysis**. Meta-analysis is a statistical method that is referred to in Chapter 5 and is not normally undertaken at undergraduate level. However, it is the principle here that is important and provides another good reason why literature reviews undertaken in this way are so useful. Undertaking a meta-analysis, or review of the results of relevant studies, has enabled researchers to establish a pattern in treatment effect that would not be apparent from reading studies in isolation.

How a literature review led to a change in practice

This was especially important in the development of the evidence base for the use of the drug Streptokinase in the treatment of myocardial infarction, which is now recognized to have saved many lives. Mulrow (1994) discusses how, in the 1970s, 33 small **clinical trials** were undertaken to compare the use of Streptokinase versus a placebo (dummy drug) in the treatment of myocardial infarction. These trials were all carried out independently and due to the small size of each trial, most did not find conclusive results in favour of the use of Streptokinase. However, these 33 trials were subsequently brought together and reviewed systematically. The results were subjected to a meta-analysis in which all the results were pooled and re-analysed. The combined results demonstrated clearly the beneficial effect of Streptokinase and, as a result, the drug became part of the standard treatment plan following myocardial infarction, thereby revolutionizing care. This review emphasized the importance of reviewing the literature systematically and the limitations of relying on any one piece of evidence. Furthermore, Mulrow (1994) identified that had this review been carried out 20 years earlier, many more lives could have been saved because evidence of effectiveness would have been available earlier.

In summary, literature reviews are important in health and social care because they enable information and research about health and social care to be viewed within its particular context and set amid other similar information and research, so that its impact can be evaluated systematically. Reviewing the literature provides a complete picture, which remains partially hidden when a single piece of research or other information is viewed in isolation. In addition, sometimes combining the results of a group of studies can lead to more convincing and useful results than the individual studies alone.

Why is there so much available information?

The amount of information available to all health and social care professionals is vast and expands on a daily basis. Every day there are media headlines, reports from conferences, reports of research from scientific journals, expert opinion followed by an opposing expert opinion. There are many reasons for this increase in information available to professionals. It is partly due to the increase in **information technology** that has led to the increasing availability of information from online journals and other websites offering information about health and social care. However, the main reason for the increase in information available within this field stems from the recent emphasis on **evidence-based practice (EBP)**, which has led to the increasing demand for research evidence upon which practice decisions should be based.

Evidence-based practice

Evidence-based practice (EBP) has been described as a new paradigm within health and social care that has gradually emerged since the 1970s. Around this time, research into health and social care gained momentum and the need to get this research into practice was recognized. Practitioners increasingly questioned their practice and searched for a scientific rationale for the care they delivered, which previously might have been given according to tradition and experience. As more and more research was carried out and the body of evidence within health and social care expanded, so did the need to apply this research into practice.

The term 'evidence-based practice' is used to refer to the appropriate application of this research knowledge to practice. Evidence-based practice has been described as the 'conscientious, explicit and judicious use of current best evidence in making decisions about the care of individual patients' (Sackett *et al.* 1996, p. 71).

Evidence-based practice involves identifying a practical question to answer and then seeking for and evaluating evidence in order to answer that question. One example of a question might be: '*Is there any evidence for the need of an all graduate nursing profession?*' The research evidence about the effectiveness and appropriateness of an all graduate nursing workforce is searched for. The **validity** or quality of that evidence is assessed and critiqued. Finally, this evidence should be applied to the context in which it is relevant; in this case, in determining policy regarding nurse preparation. Another example might be: '*What is the evidence for removing a child at risk from his or her own home?*' The research evidence that has focussed on outcomes for children at risk who have been removed from their homes, or who have remained in their homes, is then reviewed and the quality of that evidence is assessed. Finally, this evidence should be applied by those who make decisions about child welfare.

You will immediately see that sometimes this evidence can be difficult to interpret. A **research study** undertaken on one group of patients or clients may not be applicable to another. What is appropriate care for one child will not be the same as for another. However, you will also see that it is far better to use the evidence that we have than to ignore it. We cannot rely on 'gut feelings' or past experience alone when important decisions are being made. It is clear that evidence plays a vital role in determining best practice and hence in promoting evidence-based practice. However, evidence alone is rarely enough, as the above examples illustrate. An evidence-based practice approach requires that we draw on professional judgement and consider patient/client preference, *in addition to* the findings from research evidence (Aveyard and Sharp 2013).

You can now see where a literature review fits into the evidence-based practice model. A comprehensive and competently carried out literature review, which draws together all the research and other information on a topic, gives a clear picture of all the relevant studies and hence provides stronger evidence. This enables the practitioner to apply his or her professional judgement to a body of research evidence rather than to rely on one or two individual studies. This is EBP in practice!

The importance of a systematic approach to the literature review

A literature review is a vital tool because it facilitates the analysis and synthesis of research and information on a particular topic. It has already been mentioned that it is important that the review is approached in a systematic manner so that all the available information is incorporated. It has also been mentioned that when you read literature reviews, you will discover that some are undertaken in more detail than others and that the most detailed type of literature review is often referred to as a systematic review. We will now look at systematic reviews in more detail.

Systematic reviews

In its most detailed form, a systematic review strives to identify comprehensively and track down all the available literature on a topic, while describing a clear, comprehensive methodology. Systematic reviews have been defined as 'concise summaries of the best available evidence that address sharply defined clinical questions' (Mulrow *et al.* 1997, p. 389). The most well-known method for conducting a systematic review is produced by the **Cochrane Collaboration** (www.cochrane.org). The Cochrane Collaboration was established in 1993 and is a large international organization whose purpose is to provide independent systematically produced reviews about the effectiveness of health care interventions. The Cochrane Collaboration focuses mainly on systematic reviews within health care. Its sister organization, the **Campbell Collaboration**, was established to undertake and support systematic reviews within social care (www.campbellcollaboration.org).

One of the main features of a systematic review is that reviewers follow a **strict protocol** to ensure that the review process undertaken is systematic by using explicit and rigorous methods to identify, critically appraise and synthesize relevant studies in order to answer a **predefined question**. The reviewers then develop a comprehensive **search strategy**, leaving no stone unturned in the search for relevant literature, and do not regard the process complete until the search is exhausted. For example, reviewers search for unpublished research and might talk to researchers about unpublished data or articles not accepted for publication, in addition to published data on the topic in question. The reason for this is that there is evidence that a publication bias exists – that results, which show the clear benefit of an intervention, are more likely to be published than those that do not. This is especially true for studies undertaken by pharmaceutical companies, which might be reluctant to publish unfavourable results. They are, however, required by law to make the results accessible to those who request them. Thus using only published data could bias the result of the review. Reviewers then develop **inclusion and exclusion criteria** in order to assess which information they retrieve should be incorporated into the review and to ensure that only those papers that are relevant to the question(s) addressed by the literature review are included. The reviewers then *critique* the selected papers according to predetermined criteria in order to assess the quality or validity of the research identified. Studies that do not meet the inclusion criteria are excluded from the review. This is to ensure that only high-quality papers that are relevant to the literature review question are included. This process is usually undertaken by two reviewers who collaborate to ensure there is agreement about which studies are included. Finally, the findings of all the papers that are identified and incorporated for the review are pulled together and *combined* using a systematic approach. For example, a meta-analysis might be undertaken if the results of the research included in the review are reported using **statistics**, or a **meta-ethnography/meta-synthesis** can be undertaken if the results of the research included are mainly qualitative. This enables new insights to be drawn from the summary of the papers that were not available before.

The methods of undertaking a systematic review are rigorous and time-consuming. The production of a systematic review usually requires the dedication and effort of a team of experienced researchers over a period of time. Because of the comprehensive nature of the searching strategy, critique and analysis of the literature, a systematic review undertaken in the detail required by the Cochrane or Campbell Collaboration is usually considered to be the most detailed and robust form of review that exists.

Systematic reviews and clinical guidelines

In the United Kingdom, systematic reviews are used in the formulation of guidelines for the National Institute for Health and Care Excellence (NICE), whose recommendations for clinical practice are based on the best available evidence. Given the rigorous nature of Cochrane

Collaboration systematic reviews, undertaking a review in this amount of detail is beyond the means and time scales of many researchers, especially novice researchers.

Good quality (but less detailed) literature reviews

As discussed earlier in this chapter, although the stringent requirements of a Cochrane or Campbell Collaboration-style systematic review may not be within the capacity of a novice researcher, it is still possible – and indeed necessary – to undertake a 'systematic approach' to your literature review. While the term 'systematic review' is often used to refer to a review undertaken according to the Cochrane or Campbell Collaboration method of reviewing, this approach can be applied to less rigorous reviews but which have nonetheless been undertaken using a systematic and comprehensive approach. This means there can be some confusion concerning the meaning of a systematic review. One reader might interpret the term systematic review to mean nothing less than a review conducted using the methods advocated by the Cochrane Collaboration approach, while another reader might accept that a systematic review incorporates a systematic approach but may not reach the same exacting standards.

Can I achieve a systematic review in my dissertation?
Undergraduate and postgraduate students who are undertaking a literature review for their dissertation would not normally be expected to achieve a systematic review of the standard required by the Cochrane or Campbell Collaboration. They would, however, be expected to apply the general principles and guidelines of this approach to produce a literature review that uses a systematic approach in the search for critique and analysis of the literature. There is no place in health and social care for an 'unsystematic' review. For those new to literature reviewing, it is possible – indeed essential – to achieve a systematic approach to reviewing the literature, otherwise there can be no assurance that the review has been undertaken in a rigorous manner. If a literature review is to be submitted for an academic degree, the method undertaken to review the literature should always be systematic.

Narrative reviews

At the other end of the spectrum are literature reviews that are undertaken with no defined method or systematic approach. As mentioned earlier in this chapter, such reviews appear in many of the popular journals within health and social care and while they may be informative on the topic, they are likely to be biased – or not convince us that they are not biased – because the authors do not tell us how they searched for the literature included and how they evaluated it. These reviews are often referred to as **narrative reviews**. However, sometimes the term 'narrative review' is used to refer to a literature review that has been undertaken systematically but yet falls short of the rigour applied to a Cochrane systematic review. So beware the terminology used! For our purposes, the term narrative review will be taken to refer to literature reviews that do not demonstrate a rigorous method by which they were undertaken.

Narrative review   - - - - - - - - - - - - - - - - - -   Systematic review

Undefined methods of searching, critiquing and synthesizing the literature

Explicit rigorous methods of searching, critiquing and synthesizing the literature

In short, if a paper that looks like a 'literature review' does not contain a methods section, then it probably isn't a literature review.

When you come across a literature review, what is important is that you look at the method by which it has been carried out. This should be clearly stated in the methods section of the paper in which the review is written up. If a literature review does not have a well-described section in which it is clear that the researchers undertook a systematic approach to the literature review process, then you should be concerned about the quality and reliability of the findings produced. There is general concern that poorly carried out reviews do not produce reliable evidence and may be compared with poor academic practice – as described by Greenhalgh (1997), who makes reference to those who may *'browse through the indexes of books and journals until [they] came across a paragraph that looked relevant and copied it out. If anything did not fit in with the theory [they] were proposing [they] left it out'* (p. 672; my italics).

The perils of 'cherry picking' literature to include in your literature review

The following example illustrates this point. The work of Linus Pauling (1986), the world accredited scientist, who wrote a book entitled *How to Live Longer and Feel Better*, was later heavily criticized by academics who undertook further study into the area. In his book, Pauling quoted from a selection of articles that supported his opinion that vitamin C contains properties that are effective against the common cold. This book makes an interesting and convincing read. You have probably heard many people espouse the virtues of vitamin C for a variety of ailments. At first glance, Pauling's book might look like a literature review. He cites various studies and authors and all point to the positive benefits of vitamin C. However, the arguments presented in the book were challenged some years later by Knipschild (1994) among others, who undertook a systematic review of all the evidence surrounding the effectiveness of vitamin C and came to very different conclusions. He argued that Pauling had not looked systematically at all the research and had only selected articles that supported his view, while apparently ignoring those that did not. This example illustrates why such a rigorous approach is so important because, without it, your review is likely to be biased. This also explains why, when you read a report by an expert in a particular area, you should remember that his or her report represents just an expert view that might not be substantiated by evidence. This is why 'expert' opinion is generally not considered to be a strong form of evidence. Meanwhile, the debate about the use of vitamin C continues (Offit 2013).

The impact of a poorly carried out review

A poorly carried out review is one that does not use specific, identified methods for searching for, critiquing and synthesizing the literature. Instead, the methods used are often undefined and only a small selection of available literature may be incorporated in the review, which may or may not have been appraised (Hek *et al.* 2000). While some individual research papers that are relevant to the review question may be identified, if the search is not systematic, other papers may not be. The research papers that are identified are then not set in their context but remain like single pieces of a jigsaw. This may lead to a biased and one-sided review of the literature that is not comprehensive. Consequently, the conclusions drawn may be inaccurate.

How do I achieve a systematic approach to my literature review?

Whether or not you are planning to do a full systematic review, you can still undertake a systematic approach to your literature review. You should be aiming for the qualities that are inherent in a systematic review (while avoiding those inherent in a narrative approach). Think back to the structure of a literature review:

- a literature review question (or research question) set in context within an introductory chapter
- a methods section incorporating your search strategy, method of appraisal and analysis of the literature
- presentation of your results/themes incorporating critical appraisal of the studies included
- discussion of your results and recommendations for practice.

Those new to reviewing the literature are not normally expected to undertake a systematic review in the detail required by the Cochrane or Campbell Collaboration. However, you are required to undertake as systematic an approach as you can; the possible methods for achieving a systematic approach to a literature review are outlined in the subsequent chapters of this book.

Undertaking a literature review for your dissertation

This book is specifically directed towards students of health and social care who may be undertaking a literature review for the first time when they undertake their dissertation, either at undergraduate or postgraduate level. A literature review is particularly suitable for undergraduate or postgraduate students because you can undertake your review from sources that are already published and easily accessible. Undertaking a literature review does not require the formal approval of a research ethics committee, which can be a lengthy process. Students who are undertaking primary data collection (for example, interviews or questionnaires) have to submit a research proposal to their local research ethics committee, and often other regulatory bodies, for approval before they can collect their data. This process seeks to promote the safety of participants who are involved in research. The student who is undertaking a literature review is not required to obtain ethics approval prior to undertaking a review. This is because the reviewer collects data in the form of published material that relates to the research topic and then undertakes to critique and analyse the literature. The reviewer does not have direct access to those who participated in the original research and hence is exempt from seeking the approval of an ethics committee. If you are undertaking a literature review as the **dissertation** component of your degree, this clearly meets the requirements for a dissertation.

While there are many approaches to and types of dissertation, there is widespread agreement that a dissertation should meet the following criteria:

- A dissertation should be an independent and self-directed piece of academic work.
- It should offer detailed and original argument in the exploration of a specific research question.
- It should offer clarity as to how the question is answered.

A literature review meets the above criteria because a review should always commence with a research question, which is then addressed in a systematic way. It should be clearly evident that the results of the review arise from the methods used to undertake the study. The aim of a literature review is to uncover new insights on a topic by reviewing the literature in a systematic way.

This might sound an onerous task but it should not be. If you undertake your review in a systematic and comprehensive manner, you will bring together literature that sheds new light on your topic. This is not intended to sound like a daunting prospect but rather will be the result of your inquiry. Without the process of bringing together individual pieces of information to complete the jigsaw, an individual research study or other information stands alone and its real impact and relevance cannot be judged. The researcher who completes a literature review is moving from the known (the individual pieces of research and other information) towards the unknown (combining the results of the different information to reach new insights on a topic).

In summary

You should have begun to see how and why literature reviews are such an essential tool for health and social care professionals. First and foremost, they enable us to gain a comprehensive overview and summary of the available information on a particular topic. Literature reviews are generally more useful to the health and social care practitioner than any one individual piece of research because they allow one piece of research to be viewed within the wider context of others. The process of undertaking a literature review has also been introduced in this chapter. Emphasis has been placed on the importance of the literature review as a research method in its own right and its relevance as a research methodology for an undergraduate or postgraduate dissertation. We have also discussed the need to review the literature using a systematic approach in order to achieve an understanding of the body of literature as a whole in relation to a particular research area. As a general rule, when you set out to review the literature, you should aim to undertake a systematic approach as outlined in this chapter, irrespective of whether it is feasible to achieve the detail in the review as required by the Cochrane or Campbell Collaboration, for example. You can then see that if you undertake a literature review for your dissertation or research project, you are contributing to the development of knowledge in your area.

Key points

- Literature reviews are an essential tool for those who work in health and social care to make sense of the range of information that may be published on any given topic.
- Literature reviews prevent one piece of research being viewed in isolation.
- The literature review process is a research methodology in its own right and should commence with a research question, followed by a research design, presentation of results and, finally, a discussion of the results.
- The literature review process can and should be approached systematically when undertaken by a novice researcher.
- The literature review is an appropriate piece of work for a dissertation, subject to university regulations and course requirements.

2

How do I develop a question for my literature review?

- *Finding the right question for your literature review*
- *Step 1: Identify a research topic*
- *Step 2: Identify a question you can answer in your literature review*
- *Explaining the terms used in your research question and use of theory and/or a theoretical framework*
- *Reconsidering your research question*
- *Writing up the development of your research question*
- *Tips for writing up the development of your research question*
- *In summary*
- *Key points*

Finding the right question for your literature review

All literature reviews should aim to answer a specific question. You can see from the literature review process outlined in Chapter 1 that identifying a literature review question is the first step in undertaking your literature review. This might be referred to as your **research question**.

The overall aim of the question for your literature review is that, when answered, it should contribute to a better understanding of the practice area considered and ultimately improve patient/client care. However, you do not need to think that your question must be earth-shatteringly complex or sophisticated. Leave the big questions – such as what are the effects of a new drug or of the government's most recent policy on child poverty – to those with million-pound project grants and a team of highly trained researchers. Finding the right question does not necessarily mean a complex or big question. Normally the reverse is true. At undergraduate and postgraduate level, the best questions are very simple; generally they arise from your own practice and require an answer that you can feed back into practice. Finding the right question is one of the most important aspects of undertaking your literature review. We discuss this more throughout this chapter. In fact, the points made in this chapter are relevant to anyone undertaking any literature search for any purpose, even if the aim is not to write up a formal literature review.

Getting the question right

The question for your review does not have to be big but it does have to be well defined and focussed. It is very important that you develop a clear question, as without this your literature review will not be focussed. Defining a good, clear question is often difficult but it is crucial to spend time getting the question for your research right. The question provides the structure for the whole of the literature review process. A good question will act as a guide through the process of writing the literature review. It will provide a clear focus and indication as to what type of literature is required to address your question. If you get the research question right, you will find that you are directed to relevant literature that enables you to answer your question in the most appropriate way.

In contrast, if you get the question wrong – for example, if your question is vague, undefined or too broad – or indeed if you are not completely sure what question you are asking – you will find that you are unable to focus your study and are led in many different directions to an insurmountable quantity of information that is impossible to process until you finally discover that you have not actually addressed the question. A poor question will not act as a guide; if your question is vague, you will be uncertain which literature is most appropriate to use to answer the question. A question that is too broad is also unlikely to be answerable within the time frame for the writing of the review.

Avoid complex questions

An example of a question that would be too difficult and complex to answer for a small-scale project is: 'What are the effects of domestic violence on family life?' This is a huge and complex topic on which there is a lot of discussion and research evidence. Within the time span of a small-scale project, the researcher would be unable to cover the breadth of the topic and would be unlikely to be able to reach any conclusion based on the evidence reviewed. This is not to say that the researcher would be unable to comment on the issues surrounding domestic violence; however, it would be unlikely that such a big question could be addressed in a systematic manner. It would not be possible to review all the available literature and therefore the conclusions drawn would not reflect the full breadth of research and discussion. A more straightforward question might be: 'How do adolescents report the effects of domestic violence?' This question takes the larger topic of domestic violence but focuses on just one aspect of it.

Prioritize getting your question right at the beginning

Given the importance of developing a good research question that is 'do-able' within your time frame, you are advised to get your research question established as soon as you can within the time scale for your review. If your other commitments then demand your time and your literature review is put 'on hold' for some weeks or even months – as is usual for those undertaking their final year of an undergraduate degree – you can return to your review later with a firm idea about what you are intending to do. Indeed, you might find that your approach to the review has developed during the time spent on other commitments. However, if your research question is not developed by the time you are temporarily drawn away to other commitments, you will not have the assurance that you have a project that is 'do-able' when you resume your review. This could therefore delay your study.

There are two main steps you need to take when choosing the question for your literature review, which are outlined and explored below.

Step 1: Identify a research topic

Identifying your topic is necessary before you can finalize a question. For any topic, there are a good many questions that you could ask, but until you have identified your topic, you cannot identify a research/literature review question. There are a few important points to bear in mind when you are thinking about the topic you might want to explore.

Good topics and questions nearly always come from the practice environment

It is frequently the case in a practice setting that incidents arise that make you want to question your practice or the practice of others. An incident might occur that makes you keen to explore whether the optimum care/practice was carried out or whether an alternative outcome could have been achieved. It is also often the case in the busy practice environment that you do not have the time to explore incidents that arise because of other demands on your time. This is where academic study, in this case in the form of a literature review, can really complement your practice as you can use an incident that has arisen as the basis for developing your ideas for your review. This makes the literature review relevant to your professional life and a truly useful project. Your review will then be closely related to practice and you can feed your findings back to your clinical area and, indeed, when you are called to a job interview. Former students often report that they have used the expertise gained through undertaking a literature review throughout their career. It is useful to bear in mind that the ideas behind a lot of good literature reviews/research projects arise as a result of an incident that has occurred in practice that prompts the researcher to explore in more detail.

It is a good idea to 'brainstorm' a number of possible topics for your literature review. Once you have identified a possible topic, remember to keep a detailed account of the incident and include this in the introduction to your literature review, as this will set the context well for your study.

Example
A nursing student (Beed 2012) on placement in an intensive care unit recognized the challenging situation that arose when nurses were caring for patients who were potential organ donors; that is, where

patients were unconscious and at the end of their lives but their organs could potentially be used to help others. The student was aware that this was an incredibly difficult and sensitive situation for those involved in looking after these patients and identified this as a topic for her dissertation. Beed (2012) developed this topic into a research question for her literature review in which she reviewed the available evidence about nurses' experiences of this situation. From her review of nurses' experiences, she was able to make some useful recommendations. These included the need for education about organ donation, brain death and bereavement support within pre and post registration education, the crucial role of the nurse in supporting the family and continuing that role after a transplant has taken place.

Example

A social work student on a master's programme (Childs 2012) was on placement in a charity working with people with multiple and complex needs. He experienced how homeless people with mental health and substance misuse needs often seemed to struggle to access appropriate support – specifically mental health services. He experienced how both the mental health and substance misuse services expected the other service to take the lead role in care provision. As a result, individuals often seemed to struggle to access the health care they needed. From this topic, Childs (2012) identified a research question that enabled him to review the literature in this area and to make some useful recommendations. These included that further research should be undertaken into the efficacy of a dual approach to mental health and substance misuse problems and that housing should be an integral part of any intervention looking at support for homeless adults with a dual diagnosis.

You must be interested and motivated in the topic

As you start thinking about your literature review, consider aspects of your professional practice that may warrant detailed attention. As discussed above, an event that occurred in practice, for example, might trigger your interest in exploring a topic. Questions that are abstract or devised from a textbook are less likely to keep your attention or be practically useful. It is critical that the research topic you select is a topic in which you have a genuine interest.

Your literature review dissertation usually forms the most substantial component of your degree. It is a long process and will take you many months to complete. It is essential that you pick a topic in which you can maintain your level of interest. You will find that you become an expert on the topic in which your literature review is based. If you are undertaking your literature review as part of a degree, remember to prepare to discuss your topic when you attend for job interviews. It is a very good selling point for you, as it demonstrates that you have a real interest and expertise in a specific practice area. If you have selected a topic about which you are genuinely interested, you will find it easier to discuss it and might find that what becomes your extensive knowledge of this topic is helpful to you in your future career.

Once you have identified a topic, read widely

Once you have identified a possible area of interest, you are advised to read widely around the topics that interest you, in order to develop your thoughts and ideas as to which topic you would like to investigate. It is suggested that you undertake some initial literature searches in order to commence this process. Further discussion of how to search the literature is provided in Chapter 4. You will often get ideas from reading research and other papers that have already been published in the area in which you are interested. You may come across two or more studies on your topic where the results appear very different and this may prompt you to choose to review *all* the literature in this area to find out how these results fit into the literature as a whole. It is wise to ensure that the literature surrounding any potential topic is easily available. If initial searches identify literature that is located in journals that are not stocked by any library that you have access to, then your literature review will be more difficult, as you will be reliant on inter-library loans to access information. Alternatively, the literature surrounding your topic might be easily accessible but might be in journals that you do not normally access. This is not necessarily a disadvantage, however: if you select a topic that has, for example, a medical/pharmaceutical dimension, you may find that you have to negotiate and critique research methods that are unfamiliar to you.

Discuss your topic with anyone who will listen to you!

Discussing your ideas will help you clarify your own thinking in addition to getting feedback from others, for example: peers, friends, health and social care professionals, university tutors. This will help you to clarify and focus your ideas. If you have the opportunity to go to a conference or study day on an area that is closely related to your potential topic area, use this as an opportunity to discuss your ideas with others attending. If you come across research papers in your initial search for literature, email the authors and ask their advice as to which aspect of the topic they feel could be further explored through a literature review. If the topic that interests you derives from your professional practice, discuss this with those who work with you in order to get different perspectives on the topic. Discuss your area of interest with specialist health and social care practitioners working in related fields. Make contact with key people who are working in your area of interest. Explain that you are considering undertaking a project in a particular area and would like to discuss this. In most cases they will be more than happy to discuss their work with you. Even at this stage of the project, keep a diary of everything that you do: the databases you access, the libraries and keywords you use and any problems you encounter. You will need this when you come to write up the methods section of your work. You will also find the diary useful if you have to examine your own strengths and limitations and the overall limitations of the approach that you have taken.

Example of a diary

'I went to see the probation officer about support for young people when they are released from a young offenders' institution. I discussed my research ideas with him and we discussed the different agencies that are involved and what this impact may be. This has helped me to focus my question towards the role of buddies.'

Brainstorm your ideas using a mind map

You may consider using a mind map. Mind mapping is a process whereby you make notes about your ideas for a literature review question and use these to generate further ideas. In principle, mind mapping is an organized approach to developing ideas from initial ideas that you have. There are many websites available that discuss the concept of mind mapping in great detail that might be useful to access. The general principles are as follows. The main topic is written in the centre of a sheet of paper. You then identify topics that relate directly to the main topic and link these to the main topic. If there are other topics that link in but are less

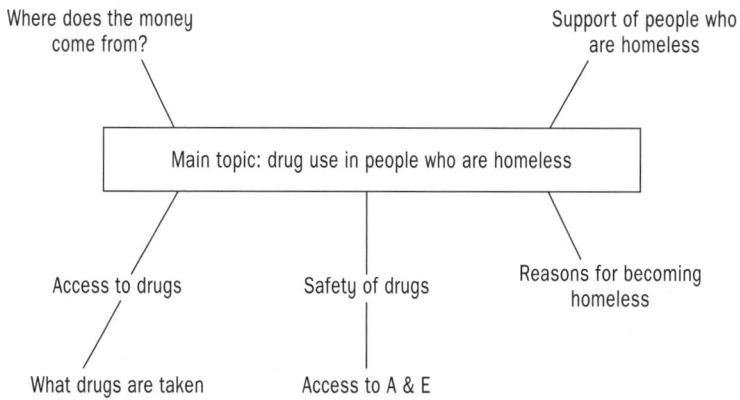

Figure 2.1 Example of a mind map

associated with the main topic, you can add another layer in your map (see Figure 2.1).

If you develop a mind map for the topic in which you are interested, you will be able to see how various aspects of the topic relate to each other and how the area you are interested in relates to the topic area as a whole. This will assist you in developing the context for your review.

From these four strategies, you should be able to identify a potential research topic. The next stage is to refine this into a manageable and workable research question on which your literature review will be based.

Consider your course requirements

If you are undertaking your literature review as a dissertation as part of a professional qualification, you need to ensure that the topic is relevant to your professional field. Most professional courses state clearly that the dissertation topic should reflect the general learning outcomes of the programme, thus it is important to develop your area of interest so that it reflects the programme that you are studying.

Example

An adult nursing student might be interested in exploring the physiological processes involved in heart disease. As this topic has a strong physiological slant, the student would be advised to adapt this to reflect an adult nursing theme. An adaptation could be to explore the role of the nurse in delivering health promotion strategies that would protect against the development of heart disease. This topic has clear relevance to adult nursing, whereas the original topic has a more physiological foundation. In almost every case it will be possible to find an aspect of the chosen topic that reflects the aim of the professional course for which the dissertation is to be submitted, especially when considering the broad knowledge base upon which professional courses are based.

If you are undertaking your literature review as part of a degree, in principle you can build on a topic that has been explored in another area of your course but do check with the university in the first instance, in case you will be penalized for repetition. It is probably reasonable to recommend that no more than 10 per cent of another module/course of study should be repeated in your literature review.

Step 2: Identify a question you can answer in your literature review

Once you have identified your research topic, the next step is to focus on a question. There are a few important points to bear in mind when you are thinking about developing your research question.

There are many possible questions that can be developed from your topic

There is the potential to develop hundreds if not thousands of possible questions from any one topic. The question you identify needs to be appropriate for your level of study; that is why it is advisable to avoid large or complicated questions.

Let's say you are a social work student and you are interested in parents' experience of looking after a child with severe learning difficulties. There are many questions that might arise from this topic. Complex questions, which are beyond the scope of a novice researcher, include: '*Is there an increased incidence of mental health problems in the parents who look after a child with severe learning difficulties?*' This is a complex question because, not only do you need to define mental health problems and severe learning difficulties, you need to consider that these might be under-reported and how you are going to recognize whether there is an increased incidence or not. You would then need to explore all the research that has examined incidence of mental health problems (as you have defined them) with looking after a child with severe learning difficulties. In addition, you would need to assess the quality of those studies and determine whether they have been undertaken with sufficient rigour to be of use to you to answer your question.

An alternative question could be: '*What is the experience of parents of looking after a child with severe learning difficulties?*', or '*Are parents able to access the help they need when looking after a child with severe learning difficulties?*' These questions are much more straightforward because, although you still need to define severe learning difficulties, you have simplified your question to an exploration of parents' experience (or their experience of finding help) rather than looking for correlations and associations between the parents' experience and the incidence of mental health problems.

Given that there are so many possible questions that can be developed from your topic of interest, the following tips will help you develop a research question that is right for you and your stage/level of study.

1. Keep your question simple and realistic to your time scale

It is probably realistic at undergraduate level, and even at postgraduate level, to have a question that is short and addresses just one question, or two at most. If you are any more ambitious than this, you are likely not to be able to answer any of the questions satisfactorily. Law (2004) has written a useful and detailed account of developing her research question, describing all the factors that contributed to the final question development. She discusses how her research question for her doctoral study was developed out of her postgraduate-level research and through discussion with those working in the area and extended reading. Clearly, for those undertaking smaller-scale projects, the question development will be a less protracted process; however, the point to be made is that the development of a question to be addressed by a literature review can be a lengthy process! Remember that your main aim is to pass your dissertation and to demonstrate that you have an understanding of the literature review process. Despite this, many literature reviews undertaken by undergraduate students *do* achieve useful insights into the research question and can lead to publication and enhance your career prospects.

2. Keep your question focussed but not too narrow

A good research question is clear and specific. The remit of the question should be small – but not too small. If the remit of the question is too big, you will be inundated with information and you will not be able to review all the information and therefore answer the question. Let's give two examples:

Example 1 – of a broad research question: *What causes cancer?*

The topic is clearly so big that it cannot be tackled by a novice researcher. Indeed, the above question is so vast that a team of researchers could explore this for a lifetime and still leave the question not fully answered! This means that it is unmanageable for a new researcher.

However, the remit of the review should not be so small that there is no identifiable literature to review! Consider the language you use to define the question. Questions beginning with 'how' and 'why' tend to lead to bigger research questions; however, if the topic area is limited, this need not make the question too broad. In general, students have a tendency to have too wide rather than too narrow a remit, so be prepared to refine the focus of your research question.

A more focussed question could be:

Example 1 – refined: *Are patients attending a GP practice aware of the importance of a healthy diet in the prevention of cancer?*

This question is more focussed and manageable. It is possible to search for evidence about patients' awareness of a healthy diet. In addressing this question, you would have to identify literature that explores patients' perception of healthy lifestyle choices.

Example 2 – of a broad research question: *What do patients think about their health or social care service?*

There are many aspects of the health or social care services in any country about which there might be research and other information, and the researcher is likely to be deluged with too much information that cannot be processed easily and systematically. Without a large research team and budget, the reviewer would be unlikely to be able to answer this question.

The following questions are more manageable:

Example 2 – refined: *What do patients think about restricted visiting times in hospital?* or *How do clients view the accessibility of their social worker?*

These questions are more focussed and address an aspect of the bigger, unmanageable question. It is possible to search for evidence on patients' perception of visiting times or the accessibility of the social work team. This literature is not likely to be extensive and should yield a manageable amount of data to appraise and critique. Any literature regarding the views of relatives and/or staff can be discounted for this review, as the remit is fixed. The only area of interest is patients' or clients' views.

3. Keep the wording of the question clear and unambiguous

The terms referred to in the question should be clear and unambiguous. You will need to define the terms in your introductory chapter so that the reader is aware of the specific remit of your work. Defining your terms will also help you to clarify exactly what you are investigating. If, for example, you are looking at a topic about the care of the older person, you need to define how you are using the term 'older person'. You need to define the terms you use – this is sometimes referred to as 'operational definitions'. You then need to make sure that you keep to this remit. It can be tempting to use interesting related literature, which is outside this remit. If this happens, you can use the literature but make sure that you change the definition of the remit of your study at the outset.

Example
If you are looking at the role of male health and social care practitioners and you come across interesting ideas that relate to female practitioners, do not be tempted to include this, except in the discussion section, unless you alter the overall remit of your study. This is discussed in greater detail in Chapter 4.

---

4. State your question as a question!

Once you have identified a question that is appropriate to your level of study and experience, think about the way your question is worded. In general, research questions can be presented as interrogative or declarative.

An interrogative question is stated as a question – for example, *'What factors affect the attrition rate of students from a university course?'*, whereas a declarative question is written as a statement – for example, *'An investigation of the reasons behind attrition rates from a university course'*.

It is recommended that you use the interrogative form when framing your research question. That is to ensure that you state a clearly defined research *question* rather than a statement. This will help to ensure that you keep your literature review focussed at all times and that all your writing is focussed on answering your question. It has already been mentioned that the research question provides the context for your entire literature review. It is therefore critical that you follow your chosen question in detail every step of the way. If your research question is phrased as a question, this will enable you to do that. It will be useful to discuss this process in depth with your supervisor.

5. Avoid leading questions

It is important to phrase your question in neutral language and to avoid phrasing your question in a leading way. As mentioned earlier, try not to make any assumptions about what you are trying to find out. Even if your research topic and question arise from a negative experience (for example, Childs 2012), and you document this in your introduction, you need to state your research question in a neutral way so that you make it clear that you are open-minded about what your answer will be. For example, in the question above about university attrition rates, we know that there is always an attrition rate from all courses so it is reasonable to look at this. However, you would need to look carefully at the litera-ture on attrition rates and write this up in your introduction as a rationale for your study.

To take another example, say your area of interest is the attitudes of professionals to young girls who seek a termination of pregnancy. You have witnessed an incident in which, in your perception, a patient was not given a good reception by staff when she presented to a clinic for a termination of pregnancy. You felt that she was left alone for a long time, with minimal attention from staff and that those who did have contact with her appeared somewhat unfriendly. You think about exploring this further. You do an initial search of the literature and do not find a lot of evidence. You consider developing a research question phrased as follows: '*How can we improve professionals' attitudes to those who seek a termination?*'

The problem with this question is that you are assuming that the atti-tudes of professionals need improving, and yet you have not found any evidence to support this, except for your observation in practice. The assumption is made that what you witnessed in the accident and emer-gency department is common practice; however, this incident might have been an isolated event and might have been because the accident and emergency department was exceptionally busy at that particular time. Therefore, it is unwise to make an assumption that professionals' attitudes need to be improved within your question, unless there is a body of evidence to back this up. While the topic is a valid and important one, it is important to phrase your question in a neutral way which does not make assumptions about practice. The question could be phrased as follows: *'What are professionals' attitudes towards those who seek a termination of pregnancy?'*

6. Remain neutral as to the possible outcomes of your review

In addition to how you phrase the question, you need to remember to keep a neutral stance to your question in your own mind. If you select a topic about which you feel very strongly, for whatever reason, you need to remain objective about your literature review from beginning to end. You must resist the temptation to pre-empt the study by having pre-drawn conclusions as to what you will find. If you find yourself wanting to prove a point, then you probably have the wrong topic – you need to remain objective. You must engage in the literature review using a systematic approach and you may be surprised by the outcomes.

7. Make sure the question is answerable using the literature

This tip is specific to those doing a literature review and may seem obvious but it does need to be considered. You need to consider whether the research question is (easily) answerable from the literature. That is, the literature must contain the information that you require to answer the question.

Example

The following is a question that could be given to students taking an advanced-level history exam: *'What were the causes of the First World War?'* The typical student will diligently access the views and arguments of leading historians and present their analysis of the causes of the war but unless they can access the primary documents on which the debate rests, they will not be able to move the discussion forward and will be reliant on **secondary sources** to address their question. In other words, they are not able to address their actual research question. The student is likely to write an extended **essay** rather than a disser-tation. However, if the question was presented as, *'What are the differing*

> views of two leading historians as to the causes of the First World War?',
> then the challenge becomes more realistic – this amended question can be
> answered using available and accessible literature, as the researcher has
> only to review the arguments presented by two leading historians. These
> arguments will be readily available. In principle, those undertaking a literature
> review should beware of literature review questions that refer to areas of
> literature that are inaccessible (for example, original documents that are not
> in the public domain), or so vast that a literature review is not manageable.

Consider the following questions:

Question 1: *What factors contribute to the use of evidence-based practice (EBP) by practitioners in social work?*

This question could be addressed by a researcher undertaking primary data collection. The question could be explored using an exploratory methodology using interviews and/or focus groups to explore these issues with the identified relevant practitioners or patients. However, it would be very different for the researcher who wanted to attempt to address these questions using literature review methodology. This is because of the availability and accessibility of the relevant material. The use of EBP is a broad topic and the researcher would have to access a very wide range of literature to identify relevant factors. Researchers would have to trawl through all the literature relating to evidence-based practice and social work in an attempt to identify factors that contribute to its implementation. This could be a very long process! Furthermore, because of this long process and the range of literature, it would be difficult to determine whether the literature had been searched comprehensively.

This question could be redefined so that it becomes manageable to the literature reviewer:

Question 1 – refined: *How do social workers refer to and implement EBP in their day-to-day activity?*

For this revised question, the search for relevant literature is more focussed. The reviewer should search for evidence of the *implementation* of EBP rather than any/all 'factors' that might contribute to the use of EBP.

Question 2: *What causes patients to self-harm?*

Similarly, the causes of self-harm are complex and this literature would also be difficult to access. There would be a lot of literature on this topic but it would be hard to find, as it is likely to be hidden within other literature and arise in many studies, but not necessarily as a main theme, and therefore is not easily identifiable.

Question 2 – refined: *What do patients who self-harm perceive to be the reasons for doing so?*

For this revised question, again the search for relevant literature is more focussed. The reviewer should search for literature concerning how patients perceive their reasons for self-harm.

8. Consider using PICOT (PICO) or SPIDER to guide the development of your research question

There are some acronyms (for example, **PICOT**, **SPIDER**) that might help you to guide the development of your research question. The letters in the acronyms refer to issues that you should consider when you develop your question. Many researchers use the acronym PICOT (as adapted by Fineout-Overholt and Johnston 2005) to guide the development of their question. The Cochrane Collaboration has adopted the use of the PICO formula (O'Connor *et al.* 2008). The prompts in the acronym are a guide to the components of a balanced and focussed research question and prompt the researcher to consider the following aspects when developing their question (please note that T is sometimes omitted from the acronym):

Population
Intervention or Issue
Comparison or Context
Outcome
Time.

Another approach is the SPIDER acronym, developed by Cooke *et al.* (2012). This new approach was designed specifically with qualitative research questions in mind and is as follows:

Sample
Phenomena of Interest
Design
Evaluation
Research.

Considering these factors within your question will help you to develop a question that is balanced and focussed. However, it is necessary to point out that using the SPIDER or PICOT acronym will not help you to develop a question unless you have ideas and a good background/rationale for a question. Thus once you have ideas for your question, consider using the SPIDER or PICOT acronym to help you refine and focus your question further.

9. Undertake some initial searches

It is very important that, as a new literature reviewer, you can determine whether a discrete body of literature is accessible in order to address the literature review question. While it is theoretically possible to undertake a systematic search of the literature, find that there is very little on your topic and write this up successfully, this is likely to be a frustrating process. Equally, it is theoretically possible to undertake a superficial overview of a vast amount of literature, in which case your critical analysis would be minimal. However, neither of these options is ideal, especially at undergraduate level, where you are likely to be assessed on the *process* you undertook. It is important to demonstrate that you carried out a systematic and comprehensive process in your review. If you have an unmanageable amount of literature, it is unlikely that you will be able to demonstrate a thorough **critical appraisal** or analysis of your literature.

For these reasons, it is better to do an initial literature search to assess the scope and variety of literature that has been written on your topic, with special regard to the amount of primary empirical data there are. This will ensure that you are likely to have enough literature to answer your question and will avoid the review becoming an extended essay. If, after carrying out an initial search, there appears to be very little literature on your topic, or if there is extensive literature, you are advised to refine your research question. As a general rule, for a small-scale project at undergraduate level, an ideal range of literature would be 6–15 *research* articles that focus on your topic. Those studying at postgraduate level will be able to utilize more literature. At this initial stage of the project it can be difficult to assess the amount of literature as you will not have undertaken comprehensive searches, but it is important to bear in mind that you do not want to be overwhelmed with literature.

10. Remind yourself (often) of your question

Once you have identified your research question, you might find it useful to write it down and stick it to your computer screen, fridge or any surface where you will regularly see it. This will ensure that you do not forget your question and that you are constantly reminded of the focus of the research question. The process of developing a research question can be a lengthy one and will be shaped by what you read and your discussions with others.

Explaining the terms used in your research question and use of theory and/or a theoretical framework

Once you have established your research question, it is important to make sure that you define what you mean by the different terms or concepts you use so that there is no possibility for confusion when others read your work. Many terms can have different meanings in different contexts and it is important that you make it clear right from the beginning the exact meaning you are referring to in your work. This ensures that both you and your readers are completely clear about what your study is about. Therefore, in your introduction, you need to explore each concept that you include in your research question. You also need to define the broader concepts within which your research question fits.

Example
If you are exploring how professionals adhere to the principles of confidentiality, you will naturally define what is meant by confidentiality and the legal and ethical implications in your introduction to your review. This introductory discussion provides background information and sets the context for your review. You are not challenging this information; you are accepting it as fact for the purposes of your literature review and using it as a basis for further study. You are therefore advised to use information that is uncontroversial in this respect.

It is essential to include this information as background literature, which sets your review in context with political initiatives and legal rulings, and so on. It allows you to demonstrate that you are aware of the academic literature that is relevant to your study, and which helps to give your study focus and pertinence. You will, for example, be marked down if there are recent developments in your area that you do not acknowledge. Your introductory discussion also enables you to define the key terms you use in your review so that your reader is clear about what you are referring to in your review and there is no ambiguity. When you then finish your review, you are likely to refer back to this initial literature and relate your findings to them. This provides structure for your review and ensures that your literature review is set within a relevant academic context.

You may consider, or be asked to consider, using a **theoretical framework** to provide a structure for your literature review. The use of a theoretical framework refers to the application of a particular theory that is relevant to the research question and to which the eventual literature review is referred. This is more focussed than applying introductory background information to your study as discussed above. Paterson *et al.* (2001) describe the use of a theoretical framework to guide the development of the research question. They argue that it assists the reviewer to define relevant concepts in the literature review research question and to identify the scope of the review.

Sometimes a theoretical framework will arise naturally in relation to the research question or even be implicit within the research question.

Example

If you were exploring the way in which informed consent is managed in patients undergoing minor surgery, the theory of informed consent would be central to your study and would form a framework around which your study could be based. The results of your literature review would be reviewed in the context of informed consent theory (Faden and Beauchamp 1986) at the end of the study. Alternatively, if you were exploring motivation for smoking cessation, you might refer to the stages of change theory (Prochaska *et al.* 1994) and apply the results of your literature to this theory in the discussion.

The incorporation of a theoretical framework into a literature review can be complex. There might not be an apparent theory upon which to frame the study and in this case it is entirely reasonable to proceed without a framework. In addition, you might find that adhering strictly to a theoretical framework restricts your review and you are less open to other literature that challenges the assumptions made in the theory. Alternatively, you might actively choose not to restrict the study to a particular framework, but rather to adopt an inductive approach without a pre-existing structure. Thorne (2001) argues that the application of a theoretical framework is not essential to any research study and might have the effect of introducing bias into the study. She argues that researchers might be led in a particular direction because of the framework that is imposed and fail to be responsive to the data that are collected.

For the purpose of a literature review at undergraduate level, students are advised that reference to a theoretical framework is not required unless it is specifically requested by the academic institution in which you are studying. If a theoretical framework is obviously apparent to you as the researcher, as described above, then the underlying theory should be discussed in relation to the research question and then referred to again when the results of the literature review are discussed. If there is no obvious theoretical framework, you should use the research question to frame your literature review. A clearly defined, unambiguous research question that is expressed in a neutral way will act as a guide to the review. Those undertaking a literature review are advised to define clearly the terms they are using in their review and to articulate clear **inclusion and exclusion criteria** for literature to be incorporated in the review. This is discussed in Chapter 4.

Reconsidering your research question

It is important to emphasize that many people refine their question as they go through the process of investigation. This can occur for many reasons. You may encounter an aspect relating to your research topic that interests you more than the aspect to which your original research question relates. You might then change your question to reflect this. You might have difficulties in finding sufficient information that addresses your research question and find more literature relating to a different aspect of your topic area. You might then change your research question so that this literature can be incorporated. This might happen when you are quite a way into your review, as it is not always possible to determine how much information is relevant to your review until you have actually read it. This is discussed in Chapter 4. For example, let's say a physiotherapist is interested in evaluating the impact of journal clubs in developing increased research awareness among practitioners. At face value there seems to be no shortage of literature that addresses this topic. However, when this literature is more closely scrutinized, it becomes apparent that there is very little that actually evaluates the impact of journal clubs. The physiotherapist then broadens the research question to explore whether there is evidence for promoting the concept of a journal club rather than exploring their impact. Reconsidering the scope and title of your research question might not be as disruptive a task as you might think – you are likely to have read widely around the area and will find that the reading you have done can be applied in a different way. If you do change the scope or focus of your research question, you need to make sure that you change the title and that the entire approach to the work reflects the reworked question.

Writing up the development of your research question

When you come to write up your literature review, you will need to chart the development of your research question, beginning with how you arrived at a topic and how you refined this into a specific question. Be specific about the progress you made and what factors influenced you in this process. For example, if a conversation with a particular person proved to be vital in developing your thoughts, you should document this and the reasons why it was influential. This section is usually included in the methods section of your literature review (for further discussion, see Chapter 8) and is normally separate from your overall introduction in which you outline the topic area in which you are interested. Remember to ensure that you define all the terms that you use within your research question at the beginning of your dissertation or project.

Tips for writing up the development of your research question

1 You need to provide a good introduction to your research question, and explain why it is important to you.

2 You need to provide context for your research question. Be prepared to discuss background information that sets your question in its practical, political or theoretical context. Refer to recent relevant government or policy publications.

3 It can be useful to introduce your research question with a description of a critical incident from your practice area that illustrates why the question is important.

4 Remember to document how your research question developed through discussion with experts, email contacts and initial literature searching.

5 Remember to justify why it is appropriate to address your research question through a review of the literature rather than another research method.

6 Once you have developed your question, pin it to the fridge or anywhere you will see it regularly to ensure you address this question.

7 Add your research question to a header or footer to your developing electronic document to help stay focussed.

8 Remind your supervisor of your research question in all correspondence – they will not necessarily remember and unless they have your up-to-date question, they will not be able to assist you as well as they might.

In summary

Developing a research question can be a difficult and lengthy process but it is important as it provides the structure for the *entire* literature review. A good research question will be focussed and unambiguous, stimulating to the researcher, relevant to their area of clinical practice and achievable within the time frame. It should also be answerable from the literature. It is always good advice to write out the research question and place it in a location where you will read it often. Put your research question as a header on your documents on your computer so that you refer to it constantly. This will help you make sure that you are still answering your question and that your question does not need to be redefined. There are three main processes in the research methodology for a literature review that need to be adhered to when developing a systematic approach to addressing the research question. These three processes are addressed in Chapters 4–6: searching for literature (collecting data; Chapter 4), critically appraising the literature (Chapter 5) and analysing your findings (Chapter 6).

Key points

- Identifying a question for your literature review is a key process in the literature review methodology.
- The idea behind the question for your review will often originate from your practice area and you should be able to feed back results to the practice environment.
- It is important to identify a topic before you can focus down on a research question.
- From any topic, a wide range of questions is possible.
- Research questions should be focussed, manageable and answerable from the available literature.
- Avoid questions that are too big, as you will not be able to answer them.

3

Which literature will be relevant to my literature review?

Which literature do I need to answer my literature review question?

Once you have established the question you want to address, you need to work out which literature you need to answer the question. This is the next vital step because you will encounter a large variety of published literature within health and social care that may or may not be relevant to your research question. It is crucial to include the most relevant literature in your review and you need to work out what this is.

It is important to note that, at this point, we are talking about the literature that you will need to answer the question for your literature review rather than any background literature that you may use in your introduction. Consider the literature review process below.

The literature review process includes:

- a literature review question (or research question) set in context within an introductory chapter, including a discussion of background literature
- a methods section incorporating your search strategy, method of appraisal and analysis of the literature
- answering your question: presentation of your results/themes, incorporating critical appraisal of the studies included
- discussion of your results and recommendations for practice.

The literature used in your introductory chapter is likely to be more varied and is used to set the scene for the project. The literature you include in your review will be specific to answering your research question. At this point, it is probably worth mentioning that you should not 'use up' the literature that answers your review question in your introduction, however tempting this might be.

The availability of information on any topic you might consider is likely to have increased in recent years due to the emphasis on evidence-based practice and the expansion of sources available on the Internet. This has the advantage that journals, which were previously difficult to access, may now be available online. There is also the potential disadvantage that there is likely to be a proliferation of websites offering information on your topic area, the quality of which will vary. This means that it is more important then ever to identify which literature is relevant for your review. It is important to remember that not all the information that you will find will be of good quality and therefore of use to you.

There are two things you need to do initially:

- identify what type of literature you need to answer your research question, and
- ensure that you can recognize it when you come across it.

Exactly what is relevant to answering your literature review question clearly depends on what your literature review question is.

Example

If you are doing a literature review, say, on users' experiences of nicotine replacement therapy, the focus of your literature will be on this experience rather than on any other aspect of nicotine replacement therapy – for example, whether this is effective in assisting people to stop smoking. Yet when you do a literature search, as we shall see in the next chapters, you will probably come across literature that addresses a wide range of issues relating to nicotine replacement therapy. It is your job to focus only on literature that is relevant to your project. We look at this in more detail throughout this book.

It is also important that you can recognize different types of literature – and what you need for your review – when you search the literature. This can be a difficult task for the novice researcher who cannot be expected to be familiar with the many different approaches to the literature and to research that might have been used to explore the topic area. Furthermore, if you are undertaking a review, you will be expected not only to recognize and understand the literature encountered, but also to review and critique it. This is discussed fully in Chapter 5. However, you will often find that one or two approaches dominate the study of a particular area and this might make the process easier. Despite this, you need to be able to identify the importance and relevance of the literature you encounter. In the next section, the different types of literature you are likely to encounter when undertaking your literature review are outlined.

Different types of literature

Wallace and Wray (2006, p. 92) have provided a simple categorization system to help you to identify the literature you have access to. It may not be completely comprehensive but it should help to get you thinking about the types of literature there are, especially in your topic area. Wallace and Wray describe how the literature you encounter tends to fall into one of four categories:

1 Theoretical literature
2 Research literature
3 Practice literature
4 Policy literature.

Theoretical literature usually means literature that describes expected or anticipated relationships about the way things happen. For example, there was a time when there was a theory that the world was flat. Then, with increased knowledge, scientists were able to work out that this was not the case and the theory was disproven. In health and social care, theories are often generated in response to evidence that has been gathered and interpreted. A theory is developed that is then refined or refuted when further evidence is obtained.

Example of theoretical literature

You have probably come across Prochaska and colleagues' (1994) stages of change model. This is a theory about the stages people go through when they anticipate a behavioural change, such as stopping smoking. The theory states that people do not adopt a behaviour change in one go; they progress through different stages of pre-comtemplation, comtemplation, preparation, action, maintenance and possibly relapse. While this theory is informed by some empirical research, it is primarily a theory about behaviour change. In fact, further to the popularity of this theory, many researchers have tested the ideas held in the theory and have challenged the idea that change is always an incremental process.

You can see the link between theory and research from the example given in the box. Someone puts together a theory; this theory is then tested through research and the theory is subsequently refined. Therefore, when you come across a theory relating to your practice, remember it is only a theory – the question you need to ask is whether there is any research evidence to reinforce the claims made in the theory. Read on . . .

Research literature generally refers to a report of a systematic investigation that has been undertaken in response to the need to answer a specific question, such as: *'How long do people tend to remain in a pre-contemplative stage when anticipating behaviour change?'*, or, indeed, *'Is there any evidence that everyone goes through the pre-contemplative stage when anticipating behaviour change?'* These questions can only be answered by observing what happens in the real world, rather than in a theory. Research studies are generally undertaken according to an accepted scientific method, which involves defining a research question, identifying a method to carry out the study, followed by the presentation of results, and finally a discussion of the results. The term **empirical research** is often used. Empirical research is research that is undertaken through the observation and measurement of the world around us. An empirical study uses observation, experience or experimentation to collect new data. Data can be collected in a variety of ways, including by **questionnaire**, interview, direct measurement, and observation.

You can recognize a research paper by the way it is structured. A research paper will state its aims and objectives and will then outline the methods by which the study was undertaken. This is followed by the results and conclusion.

Research studies might be referred to as **primary research** reports. Most primary research studies are published in subject-specific journals that will be held in your academic library, and will be available either electronically or as bound copies on the shelves. Some research might use a variety of methods, which we will discuss later. This is often referred to as **mixed methods research**. You might find that primary research is reported as a secondary source in other articles, books and even newspapers, but you will not get the full account of the research unless you go straight to the primary source. This is discussed in more detail in Chapter 5.

Practice literature is literature that is written by practitioners about their field of expertise. This comes in many different forms – expert opinion, discussion papers, debate, ethical argument, information from websites, patient information leaflets and reports of good practice. You might find some overlap between research and practice literature; that is, a lot of health and social care research is undertaken in the practice setting. The way to distinguish between research and practice literature is to look for evidence of an explicit and systematic research study that has a well-described method by which the investigation or study has been carried out. If no such method exists, then the literature is likely to be practice literature. An example of practice literature is that of Walker (2013), who described the ideal management of an undiagnosed breech birth. This paper is neither a research report nor a literature review, although Walker does refer to lots of evidence.

Policy literature is literature that tells practitioners how to act in a given set of circumstances. Policies and guidelines can be written from a local or national – or in some cases international – perspective. In an ideal context, policy is based on the results of research evidence. The research on a particular topic is reviewed and policy and guidelines are written that are based on these findings. Therefore, when you review a policy, it is useful to explore the basis on which it is written in order to find out the extent to which the policy is based on current research findings.

Wallace and Wray's (2006) classification of literature is a useful start when you are considering what types of literature to include in your review. In your introduction, you are likely to include reference to possibly all four types of literature – you might refer to a recently published policy or an incident from practice or a well-known theory. However, when you get to the main body of your review, when you answer your research question, one type of literature is likely to be most useful in answering your question and you need to know what you are looking for so that you recognize it when you find it!

Which type of literature is likely to be most useful to me?

The type of literature you will include in the main body of your review depends on your review question. However, in most instances – let's say 95 per cent of literature reviews – you will be looking for research evidence in the first instance. This is because, as we have discussed previously, most literature review questions arise from practice situations and the strongest, most reliable evidence that relates to most practice situations is research. This is because research is the comprehensive study of an area and provides stronger evidence than practice literature, which is likely to be anecdotal, theoretical and policy literature, which may or may not be underpinned by research. However, as Aveyard and Sharp (2013) argue, if an area has not been well researched, and there is little research-based information available, then practice literature, for example, or discussion pieces and expert opinion, can add a wealth of insight into the topic for the reviewer. Important information would be missed if these papers were not incorporated into a literature review, as such information adds context and insight, and depth, to the arguments that are already established. We look at this in more detail in Chapter 5.

When would I look (mainly) for research literature?

Most literature review questions are best answered by looking at research literature. You would be looking for research if, for example, you wanted to explore the experience of new mothers whose newborn children are in intensive care. You need to find research studies that have focussed on this experience. You would be looking for research if you wanted to find out if one treatment or care package was better than another in any context.

When would I look (mainly) for theoretical literature?

You might be looking for theoretical literature if, for example, you wanted to review the theories of attachment between parent and child over recent decades. In this case, the main body of your review would be focusing on these theories. Thus your review would refer to theoretical literature in the first instance. You can see that this question does not relate to the practice environment directly.

When would I look (mainly) for practice literature?

You might be looking at practice literature if you wanted to explore the ethical debate about a particular topic. Practice (or anecdotal) literature will also be relevant to many research questions but will not be as strong as research evidence.

When would I look (mainly) for policy literature?

You might be looking at policy literature if, for example, you wanted to explore the development of local policies for infection control in your review. To do this, you would need to access the relevant policy literature in the first instance.

Looking closely at your research question

You can usually tell from your research question which type of literature you need to access in order to answer it, and it is likely to be research literature. However, if it is not immediately obvious, then spend some time with your supervisor to try to identify this. Later in this chapter, we discuss how it is not only important to be able to recognize whether you need research, theory, practice or policy literature but that it is also necessary to work out what type of research is most useful to you. In order to do so, we need to explore the types of research that there are and how they help us answer particular questions.

Types of research that might be relevant to you

Given that research is likely to be the type of literature most relevant for your review in most cases (depending on your research question), we now take a closer look at this type of literature. In summary, research can be classified as follows:

Original empirical research/primary research

- Systematic reviews and good quality literature reviews
- Quantitative research
- Qualitative research
- A mixed methods approach.

Systematic reviews and good quality literature reviews

Systematic reviews and good quality literature reviews might be very relevant to the question you are answering for your literature review. Systematic reviews, which have a detailed **research methodology**, should be regarded as a robust form of evidence when they are identified as relevant to a literature review question. This is because they seek to summarize the body of knowledge on a particular topic, enabling you to see the whole picture rather than just one isolated piece of research. This means that systematic reviews are very useful summaries of existing evidence. However, given that your task as a student is to undertake a literature review, you need to consider carefully any systematic or good quality literature reviews you come across, as these might well answer your research question and leave you with little more work to do, which might hinder your chances of satisfying your examiners! We will discuss how you manage existing literature reviews in later sections of this book.

Quantitative research

Quantitative research, sometimes referred to as positivist research, uses experimental methods and/or methods that involve the use of numbers in the collection of data. Traditionally, there is no involvement between the researcher and participant, and the researcher stands metaphorically 'behind a glass screen' to conduct his or her research. The studies tend to involve many participants and the findings can be applied in other contexts.

Example

Quantitative experimental methods have been used to explore whether a lumpectomy is better than a mastectomy in the treatment of breast cancer. Clinical trials were conducted comparing the two treatment options and the results (survival outcomes) were measured numerically in months and years. The researcher divided the participants into two groups, allocated the treatment and observed the outcomes. In principle, quantitative researchers seek causal determination and predictability. Quantitative research is appropriate only in cases when data can be collected numerically; for example, the number of 'disease-free years' experienced by a patient, or the number of days for a wound to heal using one dressing or another.

Types of quantitative research

Some of the different types of quantitative studies, and when you might use them in your review, are described below.

Randomized controlled trials

Randomized controlled trials (RCTs) are a form of clinical trial, or scientific procedure, used to determine the effectiveness of a treatment or medicine. Therefore, if your literature review question is asking *whether something is better than something else* or *whether something is effective or not,* then RCTs are what you need to look for in the first instance. They are widely considered to be the 'gold standard' for research in which it is desirable to compare one treatment with another (or no treatment). In an RCT, participants are placed by random allocation into two or more groups. To illustrate this most easily, let's say that participants are allocated into just two groups. An intervention is then given to all participants in the first group but not to participants in the second. At the end of the trial, the different outcomes of the participants in the two groups are compared. The researcher is looking for differences between the different treatment groups of the trial that can be attributed to the intervention. It is common for one of the groups to be a control group who receive standard treatment or a placebo group who receive no treatment. A placebo group is, however, only ethical if non-treatment is not thought to be harmful to participants, such as if there was genuine uncertainty as to the effectiveness of a treatment.

Randomization – or chance allocation – into an experimental group

The important feature of an RCT is that the participants are allocated into the different treatment groups of the trial at random. The process of **randomization/random allocation** is equivalent to the tossing of a coin. The process ensures that participants are allocated into the different groups by chance rather than by the expressed preference of the patient or researcher. It is very important that neither the participant nor the researcher has any control over the group to which a participant is allocated. This is because the researcher is looking for differences between the treatment groups of the trial that can be attributed to the intervention. This can only be determined if the different groups – commonly referred to as 'arms' – of the trial are essentially equal in all respects except from the treatment given.

It is important not to confuse the process of randomization/random allocation used within an RCT with the concept of **random sampling**, which is discussed later in this chapter.

The reason random allocation is important is as follows. If the research participants were to choose which treatment group of the RCT they wanted to enter, it is very likely that one particular treatment group would be more popular than another and the different treatment groups in the trial would not be equal. Let's say that researchers wanted to explore a new drug for helping people to stop smoking. They need to allocate participants by random assignment into one of two treatment/control groups of the trial. If either the researcher or participant had been allowed to choose who should go in each group, those more committed to quitting might have chosen the arm of the trial with the new drug and those who were less committed might have chosen the arm of the trial with the dummy tablet (placebo). The two treatment groups of the trial would then not be equal. It would then not be possible to determine whether the differences in outcomes observed between the different treatment/control groups of the trial were due to the new drug or whether they were due to the differences in the characteristics of the participants who had self-selected into one group or another.

If it is particularly important that participants with specific characteristics are equally represented in both groups (for example, those with young children might have different smoking habits from those without children and you might want an equal number of these participants in each group), then a further form of randomization can be used called **stratification** (or minimization), in which a computer-generated process allocates an equal number of people who have or do not have children into each group. This is an additional statistical process that assists in ensuring that the groups are equal in respect of certain predefined criteria that are relevant for the research.

Once each treatment group in the trial has been randomly allocated, the groups are considered to be equal, and the intervention treatment is given to the first group. The second group receives either the standard treatment (or no treatment or placebo, depending on the individual study design). The groups are then observed and the differences between the groups in terms of smoking cessation rates are monitored. Given that the two groups of participants were randomly allocated and hence can be considered to be 'equal', any difference in smoking cessation rates between the groups can be attributed to the effect of the drug. A 'null' hypothesis is usually stated when an RCT is designed. The **null hypothesis** states that there is no difference between the two groups. The aim of the RCT is to determine whether the null hypothesis can be confirmed or rejected. If the results show that there is a difference between the control group and the intervention group, then the null hypothesis can be rejected. A flow diagram of the process of conducting a RCT is presented in Figure 3.1.

RCTs are considered to be one of the best forms of evidence when looking at the effectiveness of treatment. You should look for RCTs in the first instance if your question is seeking to establish whether something is effective or not. RCTs are undertaken in all areas of health and social work. However, if it is not possible to randomize participants in a research study and expose one group to a particular procedure, then it is

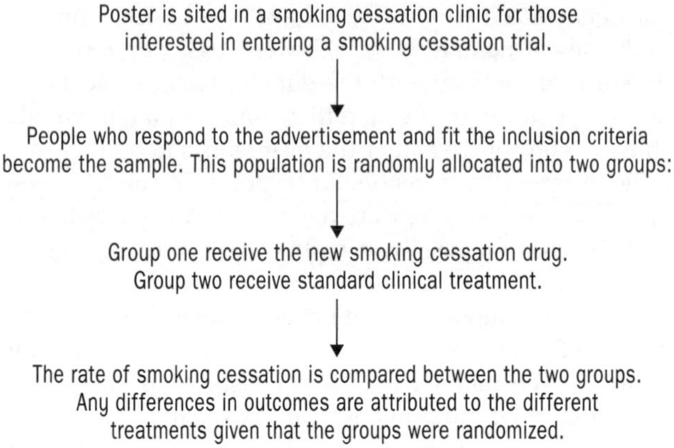

Poster is sited in a smoking cessation clinic for those
interested in entering a smoking cessation trial.

↓

People who respond to the advertisement and fit the inclusion criteria
become the sample. This population is randomly allocated into two groups:

↓

Group one receive the new smoking cessation drug.
Group two receive standard clinical treatment.

↓

The rate of smoking cessation is compared between the two groups.
Any differences in outcomes are attributed to the different
treatments given that the groups were randomized.

Figure 3.1 The process of conducting an RCT

not possible to carry out an RCT. Thus, the RCT is only one of many
approaches to research that might be useful in addressing your research
question.

Example
Question: *'Is it better to treat people at the site of an accident or take them to
A&E as soon as possible?'* For this question, you would need to search for
randomized controlled trials that explored the effectiveness of roadside care
versus immediate hospital care.

Cohort and case control studies

Cohort studies and **case control studies** are both types of
observational study. These studies attempt to discover links between
different factors and are often undertaken when it is not possible to
carry out an RCT. They have often been used to find the causes of
disease.

A cohort study is the study of a group of people who have all been
exposed to a particular event or lifestyle (for example, they all smoke).
They are then followed up in order to observe the effect of the exposure
to smoking nicotine on their health and well-being.

Seminal work using cohort studies

One of the most famous cohort studies, which took place in the 1950s, followed up a group of people and was able to demonstrate that smoking causes lung cancer. At this time, smoking was considered normal and harmless and a large percentage of the population smoked. Many people thought that pollution was the cause of lung cancer. Smoking was not considered to be a risk factor. The epidemiologists, the late Sir Richard Doll and Bradford Hill (1954), conducted a cohort study in which they followed up a group of doctors, some who smoked and some who did not. They then observed this cohort to determine whether those who smoked were more likely to develop lung cancer than those who did not. This cohort study demonstrated that there was a strong association between smoking and lung cancer.

A flow diagram of the process of conducting a cohort study is presented in Figure 3.2.

A case control study is one in which patients/clients with a particular condition are studied and compared with others who do not have that condition, in order to establish what has caused the condition in the original patients/clients.

Case control study

Doll and Hill (1954) also carried out a case control study examining lung cancer patients and traced back to see what could have caused the disease. They designed a questionnaire that was administered to patients with suspected lung, liver or bowel cancer. Those administering the questionnaire were not aware of which of the diseases was suspected in which patients.

It became clear from the questionnaires that those who were later confirmed to have lung cancer were also confirmed smokers. Those who did not have lung cancer did not smoke. Clearly, it would not have been possible to have undertaken an RCT to explore the causes of lung cancer as it would not have been possible to randomize a group of non-smokers and ask one group to start smoking! It is therefore appropriate to use case control studies and cohort studies to explore relationships between different variables if an RCT is not possible.

Cohort of people who all experienced the same exposure/experience.

This cohort is followed up to observe the effect of this exposure.

They may be compared to a control group who did not experience this exposure, but because the groups were not formed by random allocation, any observed differences between the two groups at the end of the study period are not as easily attributable to the exposure as if the study has been an RCT.

Figure 3.2 The process of conducting a cohort study

A flow diagram of the process of conducting a case control study is presented in Figure 3.3.

When would I need cohort and case control studies?
You might be searching for cohort and case control studies when you are looking for causation and associations between different variables, especially when a RCT has not been possible. For example, for the question, 'Are parents of children with attention deficit disorder more likely to be diagnosed with depression?' For this question, you would be looking for case control and cohort studies which explore the incidence of depression in parents with and without a child with attention deficit disorder.

Cross-sectional studies (surveys/questionnaires)

Surveys and questionnaires are studies in which a **sample** is taken at any one point in time from a defined population and observed/assessed. A cross-sectional study could be used to assess illicit drug use in a university population, for example. This could be undertaken by the use of a questionnaire or survey, although their use is by no means limited to this

Individuals with a specific condition or situation are identified.

The circumstances that led up to the development/progress of this condition are then explored.

Figure 3.3 The process of conducting a case control study

research approach. Questionnaires/surveys are printed lists of questions used to find out information from people. They can be used as a means of data collection in RCTs, cohort and case control studies, and are often used to find out specific information from people at one point in time only.

Quality in questionnaire design and administration

The development of a questionnaire is an arduous process and the information obtained is highly dependent on the quality of the questionnaire developed. There are many potential pitfalls: a long questionnaire might be discarded by the respondent before completion, while complicated or badly worded questions may be misunderstood by the respondent. Postal questionnaires have the additional disadvantage that there is likely to be a low response rate. If large sections of the target population do not respond, the overall quality of data collected will be poor. Questionnaires that are administered in a face-to-face interview will generally result in a higher response rate. A thorough exploration of the use of questionnaires in research is given by Oppenheim (1992). In an ideal questionnaire survey, a well-designed and piloted questionnaire is administered to an appropriate sample and the response rate is high.

The purpose of a cross-sectional study is to provide a snapshot illustration of the attributes of a given population in the sample; for example, to explore the incidence of illicit drug use at one point in time. The nature of the questions asked can provide descriptive data, for example: '*How many university students use illicit drugs on campus?*' Alternatively, some further analysis can be attempted, for example: '*Do all those who report using Class A drugs also report early illicit drug use?*'

However, data obtained from a questionnaire study are always limited by the following factors. First, it is often not possible to obtain access to an entirely representative sample for the distribution of a questionnaire, nor is it likely to achieve a complete response rate to the questionnaire/survey. Thus, the completed questionnaires will contain information from a selection of, but not a random sample of, students and will therefore give an incomplete picture of illicit drug use. Second, any apparent associations arising from the analysis of questionnaire data should be interpreted with caution. For example, if it was identified that those who used illicit drugs also experienced high anxiety levels, it would be tempting to conclude that the use of illicit drugs increases student anxiety. However, perhaps the reverse is true and that those with high levels of anxiety resort to illicit drug use. It is very difficult to determine relationships between variables in a questionnaire/survey.

When would I need cross-sectional studies?
You are likely to use cross-sectional studies for measuring specific actions, attitudes and behaviours of a given group of people, such as for the question, '*What do students report about their experience at university?*' For this question, you are expecting to get a broad range of students' reports and you would therefore be looking for questionnaires and surveys which had explored this.

Random sampling and quantitative data analysis

Quantitative research sometimes uses random sampling. This means that the sample is picked at random from the overall population. Random sampling is generally defined as meaning that all those in the sample have an equal chance of being selected in the sample. This is important because it ensures that the sample is not biased. For example, a random sample of university students could be drawn from the university admissions list rather than from attendance at lectures, given that all students will be on the admissions list, but not all will attend lectures. Any sample drawn from those who attend lectures will be biased rather than random. It is important to note that obtaining an unbiased sample in any research study is very difficult. A questionnaire might be sent to a random sample of the population, but unless there is a 100 per cent response rate, the responses obtained will be biased. It is also important to note that some studies use random allocation within a non-random sample, rather than random sampling overall. An RCT, for example, will normally have a convenience sample from which two or three random groups are composed. When you are reviewing a quantitative study, be aware of the sampling strategy and be able to comment on the reasons as to why this approach has been adopted. Consider whether a random or non-random sample was used and whether this was appropriate.

Statistics

Quantitative data analysis is generally done using statistics. There are two types of statistics. First, there are **descriptive statistics** that describe the data given in the paper. These statistics should describe clearly the main results – for example, how many people answered 'yes' to a particular question, or what the most common response to a question was. The average answers will typically be given using the mean, median and mode responses. The data should be clearly described so that you can identify the main findings of the paper.

Second, there are **inferential statistics**. The purpose of inferential statistics is to **generalize** to the wider population. In other words, to determine the extent to which the data obtained from a sample are representative of the wider population as a whole. Inferential statistics provide a means of drawing conclusions about a population, using the data obtained from a sample taken from that population. For example, if you have a questionnaire survey of 1000 people, of which 500 stated a preference for holidaying abroad, inferential statistics can be used to determine whether this result would be accurate for the whole population, rather than just this sample. Inferential statistics do more than describe a sample; they infer from it to the wider population. The bigger the sample, the more certain you can be that the sample prevalence is close to the population prevalence.

Confidence intervals

The confidence we can have that the sample is an accurate indication of the true population prevalence is reflected in **confidence intervals**, which give numerical limits to a 'common-sense' approach. Confidence intervals are used to estimate the confidence that the sample reflects a range within which the true score is known to lie. The smaller the interval or range, the more confident you can be that the results in the study reflect the results you would find in the larger population. Using a formula, the confidence intervals – upper and lower – are calculated. A 95 per cent confidence interval means that we can be 95 per cent sure that the true population prevalence lies between the lower and upper confidence interval.

Example

100 students are asked to document the number of hours per week spent using a mobile phone. The mean number of hours is 4. The confidence intervals are calculated as 2.5–5.6. This means that you can be 95 per cent confident that students spend between 2.5 and 5.6 hours per week using a mobile phone.

P-values

Statistics are often described as a **P-value** or probability value. The *P*-value expresses the probability of the results shown in the paper being due to chance. *P*-values test a **hypothesis**. They remove the 'best guess' that the results found are not due to chance. It is important to determine the play of chance in any research. Let's say you are undertaking an RCT and have two randomly allocated groups, A and B. Normally in an RCT, you would give an intervention to one group and not to the other and then examine the differences in outcomes between the groups. However, let's say that on one occasion no intervention was given. Both groups were treated with the standard treatment. Yet, when you examine the outcomes in each group, you will inevitably see a variety of outcomes in each group, due to natural differences between the groups, even though both groups were given the same treatment. Now let's say that you do then administer an intervention to one of the groups and observe the different outcomes of the two groups. The *P*-value can then be calculated to determine whether the difference in outcomes observed is due to chance. To calculate the *P*-value we use the null hypothesis. The null hypothesis states that there is no relationship between the variables under study. The *P*-value expresses the probability of the results occurring, if the null hypothesis were true; that is, if no relationship was found. This can be calculated using a statistical test, for example the chi-squared test. A *P*-value of 0.05, for example, means a 0.05 (1:20) chance of seeing these results if the null hypothesis were true. This means it is unlikely that the null hypothesis is true and that there is a relationship between the variables. It is important to remember that this does not indicate a causal relationship – that is, that one variable caused the other – but just that the two occur together.

Example

Take the following hypothesis. Students who get a 2:1 degree are more likely to enter clinical management than those who get a 2:2. The null hypothesis is that there is no difference in degree outcome in those entering management. In a study of 100 students, 30 students obtained a 2:1 and entered management, and 20 students obtained a 2:2 and entered management. The chi-square test showed a *P*-value of 0.2, which means there is a one in five chance that these results were due to chance rather than the effect of degree classification.

Risk ratios and odds ratios

Differences between two or more groups in a RCT are often expressed as a **risk ratio** or **odds ratio**. To understand these terms, consider a study that explored the effect of a new intervention to help people stop smoking. In the intervention group, 40 out of 100 people stop smoking. In the control group, only 20 out of 100 people stop smoking. To calculate how much more likely you are to stop smoking if you take the new intervention, we take the proportion of people who stop with the new drug (40/100) and divide by the proportion of people in the control group who stop (20/100). The answer is 2 and we can say that people are twice as likely to stop smoking if they use the intervention. This figure is the risk ratio. (The odds ratio is slightly less intuitive and is not often used for reporting trials and is defined in the glossary.) RCTs can only be used when it is possible to allocate participants within a group at random and administer a treatment or intervention to one group and not to the other. When this cannot be done, often for ethical reasons, a modified experiment may be considered.

How much understanding of statistics do you need?

The simple answer is that it is important that you understand what the results of the studies mean, rather than have a detailed understanding of what the actual statistics used in the studies mean. So when you read a study, make sure you can understand, in general terms, what the researchers are trying to do – for example, are they aiming to compare the difference between two groups who have had different treatments or care programmes, or to work out whether there is an association between one group and another? Before you try to understand the statistics, make sure you are clear about the aim and purpose of the study. When the statistics are presented, together with an interpretation of the results, you will find these easier to understand if you have an understanding of the purpose of the paper.

Qualitative research

In contrast to quantitative studies, **qualitative research** is concerned with exploring meaning and phenomena in their natural setting. This research is sometimes referred to as 'naturalistic research'. Researchers seek to understand the entirety of an experience. For example, qualitative researchers might explore what it is like for a patient to be diagnosed with breast cancer in order to ensure that adequate support is available to such women. These data are not numerical but are collected, often through interview, using the words and descriptions given by participants. The data are used to generate understanding and insight of the situation being researched. There is no (or little) use of statistics in qualitative research; the results are descriptive and interpretative. Some researchers argue that qualitative research is non-generalizable because it is context-specific; however, it is has been broadly accepted for at least a decade that the insights and interpretations gained from qualitative enquiry are generalizable and can be transferred from one setting to another (Morse 1999). Therefore, if your literature review question is seeking to answer a question that requires this rich data, you are likely to be looking for qualitative studies.

The fundamental principle of all qualitative approaches is to explore meaning and develop understanding of the research topic. There are a wide variety of approaches to qualitative research (Shin *et al.* 2009). **Qualitative data** are often collected through the descriptions and words of those participating in the study rather than by numerical measurement as in quantitative research. For this reason, qualitative approaches often use in-depth interviews as the main type of data collection, as this allows thorough exploration of the topic with the research participant. Other means of data collection include focus groups and direct observation. The sample, or participants used in a qualitative study, tends not to be selected at random, as is often the case with a quantitative study; instead, participants are selected if they have had exposure to or experience of the phenomenon of interest in the particular study.

Purposive sampling

This type of sampling is referred to as **purposive sampling** and this leads to the selection of information-rich cases, which can contribute to answering the research question. Sample size tends to be small in a qualitative study, due to the need to develop an in-depth understanding of a particular area. This is because researchers are seeking to develop insight into the topic area and a small number of participants who can provide 'information-rich' data is more important than a larger sample from whom the data would not be so insightful.

Qualitative data are usually analysed using the whole text. There are various ways of analysing qualitative data, but most of the approaches involve transcribing recorded interviews, assigning a named code to each section of the transcribed data and then ordering (making sense of) these codes to form categories. These categories are then used to build a description of the results. One of the attributes of qualitative research is that when researchers analyse the data, they do not impose their own preconceived ideas onto the data set. They do not set out looking for specific ideas, hoping to confirm pre-existing beliefs. Instead, they code the data according to ideas arising from within it. This process is often referred to as *inductive*. However, qualitative research is by its nature a subjective enterprise. Researchers do not generally strive to achieve objectivity because this would strip away the context from the topic of research. Furthermore, the researcher cannot achieve complete objectivity because he or she is the data collection tool (for example, the interviewer) and interprets the data that are collected. This is acknowledged in the research process and steps are taken to maintain objectivity as far as possible.

Types of qualitative research

There are many types of qualitative research. Many are described in the literature generically as 'qualitative studies' and are not sub-defined further. However, there are some specific approaches to qualitative research that are further defined. These are outlined below. You need to be able to identify and recognize these different approaches to qualitative research and to understand why one approach was selected for a specific research question.

Grounded theory was one of the first qualitative research approaches to be documented by the social scientists Glaser and Strauss (1967). The purpose of grounded theory is the systematic development of a theory from a set of data that are collected for the purposes of the research. Here again, you can see the link between theory and research. In grounded theory, data are often collected using interviews and observations. The specific components of grounded theory that must be incorporated into a study include:

- **theoretical sampling**, in which the sample is not preset but is determined according to the needs of the ongoing study

- constant comparison analysis, in which data are analysed as they are collected and constantly compared with other transcripts
- saturation, in which data collection ceases only when the data analysis process ceases to uncover new insights from the data.

Phenomenology is the study of lived experience, or consciousness. Literally, phenomenology is the study of 'phenomena': the appearances of things and the meanings things have in our experience. Therefore, in a phenomenological study, the research topic is studied from the point of view of the lived experience of the research participant. These studies often use in-depth interviews as the means of data collection, as they allow the participant the opportunity to explore and describe the lived experience within an interview setting. If your literature review question is looking at patient or client experience of a situation, you are likely to be looking for phenomenological studies in the first instance.

Ethnography is the study of human social phenomena, or culture. An ethnographic study focuses on a community in order to gain insight into how its members behave. Participant observation and/or in-depth interviews may be undertaken to achieve this. Ethnographers typically carry out first-hand observation of daily behaviour (for example, how health care professionals act in a hospital setting) and may even participate in the actual process as a participant-observer. Ethnography is fieldwork-based and seeks to observe phenomena as they occur in real time. A true ethnographic study is a time-consuming process.

Action research, or collaborative enquiry, is the process by which practitioners attempt to study their problems scientifically in order to guide, correct and evaluate their decisions and actions. Action research is often designed and conducted by practitioners who analyse the data to improve their own practice. This research can be done by individuals or by teams of colleagues. The advantage of action research over more traditional approaches to research is that it has the potential to generate genuine and sustained improvements in organizations. These improvements are not imposed on institutions in the form of research findings, but are generated as solutions from within.

When would you use qualitative research?

You would use qualitative research when your research question is exploratory rather than seeking to measure something, for example:

- *What are women's experiences of a refuge centre?*
  For this question, you would be looking at explorative studies of women's experiences, for example, phenomenological studies.

- *Why do students experiment with illicit drugs?*
  For this question, you would be looking for qualitative studies that explored the reasons why young people use illicit drugs, and this might be explored in ethnographic, phenomenological or grounded theory studies.

The merits of quantitative and qualitative research

There has been much debate in the research literature about the relative merits of both quantitative and qualitative research, with some researchers proclaiming the superiority of one approach over another. It is evident from our discussion about the different research approaches that these debates are not important. What is important is that the most appropriate research methodology is used to address the research topic in question. There are many similarities between the two approaches to research. Both commence with a research question and select the appropriate methodology to answer this question. In all research papers, the methods used to undertake the research should be clearly explained and the results clearly presented.

The research methods outlined above are just some of the methods that you might encounter when you undertake a literature review. In addition, many researchers now use a 'mixed methods' approach where different methods are used to address one research question. It is important that you are familiar with the different approaches to research design so that you can appraise the quality of the literature that is to be incorporated in the review. This is discussed in greater detail in Chapter 5.

Mixed methods research

The research methods outlined above are just some of the methods that you might encounter when you undertake a literature review. In addition, many researchers now use a 'mixed methods' approach where different methods are used to address one research question. For example, a researcher might use both qualitative and quantitative approaches to explore a research question or topic from different perspectives. Qualitative approaches can be used to add depth and insight to the findings of a quantitative study. Alternatively, quantitative approaches can be used to verify the findings of a qualitative study. It is therefore important that you are familiar with the different approaches to research design so that you understand the various approaches that might be included in any one piece of research.

The use of secondary sources

A secondary source is a source that is a step removed from the ideas you are referring to. Secondary sources often comment on primary sources. For example, a report in the *British Medical Journal* (BMJ) might refer to a systematic review published by the Cochrane Collaboration. The BMJ report would be the secondary source and the Cochrane Collaboration report, the primary source. You are advised to access the primary source wherever possible and the use of secondary sources should be avoided throughout a literature review. This is because if you rely on a secondary report and you do not access the original report, there is a margin for error in the way in which the primary source was reported.

For example, let's say that the author of a paper you are reading (author 1) cites the work of another author (author 2) who has done work in the area. If you refer to the work of author 2 without accessing the original work, this is a secondary source and should be avoided when you are undertaking a literature review. This is because in a literature review you are striving for authenticity. Unless you read the original work by author 2 directly, you are relying on another author's report of this work. This means that you cannot comment on the way it is represented by author 1 or the strengths and limitations of this work.

It is an important part of the literature review process that you identify the context in which the information is written, so that you are not misled by the way in which the reference is cited. It is easy to see how an author (for example, author 2) can be misquoted in a paper written by another author (here, author 1). If this paper is then cited by author 3, author 2 can be further misquoted. Bradshaw (2001) provides a good illustration in her historical account of the influences of modern-day nursing of how secondary sources have been used to inform influential government reports and how this has led to misleading conclusions. Therefore, where you need to quote an author directly, you are always advised to access this paper rather than to refer to a report of this paper, unless it is not possible to get hold of the primary source; for example, if it is out of print or an unpublished doctoral thesis. For this reason, you should avoid using secondary sources throughout your literature review.

Is one type of evidence better than another?

The term **'hierarchy of evidence'** means that some forms of evidence are stronger than others in addressing a specific type of literature review question. When you are doing a literature review, this concept is very important as you need to make sure you use the strongest evidence to answer your literature review question. Simply put, research evidence is generally stronger evidence than anecdotal evidence and research evidence would therefore be further up the hierarchy. But it is not this simple, as different types of research are better for some literature review questions than for others. Therefore, there is not just one hierarchy of evidence, as we shall see below. What amounts to strong evidence for one literature review question will not be the strongest evidence to answer another – just as there are many different questions, so there are many different hierarchies of evidence. It all depends on your literature review question. In any hierarchy of evidence, the higher up a methodology is ranked, the more robust it is assumed to be.

There are a variety of hierarchies of evidence that have been developed to guide you towards the evidence that is strongest for your particular literature review question. One of the first hierarchies of evidence, developed by Sackett *et al.* (1996), is for ranking the strength of evidence to show how effective a treatment or intervention is. This hierarchy of evidence *for determining effectiveness* goes in the following order:

1 Systematic reviews of RCTs
2 RCTs
3 Cohort studies, case-controlled studies
4 Surveys
5 Case reports

6 Qualitative studies
7 Expert opinion
8 Anecdotal opinion.

So, for literature review questions, when you want to find out whether or not something is effective – in either health or social care settings – this is the hierarchy you would use. You would look for systematic reviews in the first instance followed by RCTs. These would be the most important studies in your review followed by studies further down the hierarchy.

Example
Imagine you are a midwifery student and your question for your literature is whether one type of epidural is more effective than another. To answer this question, the best evidence will be studies that have compared one epidural directly with another (RCTs). Therefore, a systematic review of RCTs that compared different types of epidurals, or individual RCTs, would provide stronger evidence than a qualitative study that asked the opinion of mothers as to how they experienced the epidural. This is not to say that the opinion of mothers in unimportant but for an objective assessment of whether one epidural is better than another, a study that compares both in a systematic way provides stronger evidence. The stronger evidence provided by the RCT in this instance indicates that the RCT should be placed higher up in a hierarchy of evidence than a study exploring mothers' experience of pain relief *when addressing this particular question*.

However, if you wanted to know how mothers felt about receiving an epidural, then a qualitative study that explored this in depth would be more useful than a RCT comparing different epidurals for *addressing this particular question*.

Why do some literature reviews include predominantly RCTs?

Traditionally, the Cochrane Collaboration was established to increase our knowledge base concerning the effectiveness of treatments and care procedures. And, as we have seen above, we need RCTs to find out if something is effective or not. This applies to all aspects of health and social care, although sometimes it is not possible to undertake a RCT. For example, Faggiano *et al.* (2006) published a review that evaluates the effectiveness of school-based interventions in improving the knowledge of schoolchildren regarding illicit drug use. In this review, the authors incorporated all the available RCTs that compared one school-based intervention for illicit drug use with another in order to determine which interventions were most effective overall.

But not all literature review questions are about 'finding out what works best'

In recent years, literature reviews have been used to evaluate far more than the effectiveness of treatments or interventions. And for literature review questions that *do not* seek to evaluate the effectiveness of a treatment or intervention, RCTs will not be the best or only evidence to use. We have reviewed the different types of research and it is clear that while RCTs are useful in determining effectiveness, they cannot provide evidence regarding all other aspects of care within health and social care. For questions not concerned with effectiveness of treatments or interventions, there are more appropriate ways of collecting data that will help you address the literature review question. For example, researchers concerned with exploring client experience of day care services would be likely to explore this through interviews with the clients themselves rather than to conduct a trial to explore the differences between two types of intervention. For these reasons, there is increasing recognition that systematic reviews should seek to incorporate the types of research that are most likely to address the research question, rather than limit their inclusion criteria to RCTs. There is now general acceptance that all types of literature can, and indeed should, be included in a review if it is relevant to the review question.

Working out which evidence you need for your literature review

It is important to look closely at your research question and work out which literature is most relevant for your own review. In health and social care, and especially in the research questions that arise from the practice environment, knowledge is obtained from a variety of different sources and many different types of research contribute to our under-standing of a wide range of situations encountered in everyday practice in health and social care. It is therefore appropriate to say that the most robust form of evidence for addressing a particular research question will be determined *by that research question*.

Identifying your own 'hierarchy of evidence' in your review

For this reason, when you design your literature review, you are encour-aged to develop *your own hierarchy of evidence*, a term developed in the first edition of this book (Aveyard 2007). Your own hierarchy of evidence is based on the evidence you need to address your particular question. Every literature review question will require different literature to address it most effectively. Therefore, you need to think carefully about the type of evidence you need to address your research question and run your ideas by your peers and, of course, your research supervisor. To get you started, you might like to consider in very simple terms whether your question will be addressed best using qualitative or quantitative research or a combination of both.

Example A: When experiments are the best evidence

Imagine you are doing a literature review exploring the effectiveness of a particular treatment or care intervention. Let's say your review question is, '*How effective are anti-bullying policies in preventing bullying behaviour in school age children?*' In this case, the most useful literature to you will be RCTs. This is because if you want to find out whether something works or not (in this case the anti-bullying policy), you need to compare the levels of bullying where this policy has been implemented and where it has not. This is the 'gold standard' way to find out if something really works or not because of the comparison that is possible between the intervention and control group, as discussed earlier. You should therefore have RCTs at the top of your hierarchy. These are likely to provide the best and most reliable evidence with which you can address your question. However, that is not to say that RCTs are the only type of literature you should seek to identify. It might be that RCTs were not an appropriate method for exploring the topic area you have identified and you do not find any. Lower down in your hierarchy you would probably put cohort studies or case control studies that provide appropriate evidence. You would need to explore which types of studies are most suitable for addressing your research question. Evans (2003) identifies that RCTs provide strong internal validity for a study; that is, the difference in outcomes between the two groups is highly likely to be attributable to the intervention due to the controlled nature of the study. However, because of the strict protocols for inclusion in the study, RCTs are usually carried out on select groups of patients or clients who qualify for inclusion. Observational studies such as cohort studies and case control studies are less well controlled and are therefore likely to provide greater external validity; that is, the results have greater generalizability because the studies observe what is happening in practice. However, because the groups are not randomly allocated, it is not possible to determine whether differences in out-come between groups are due to the intervention.

For example A, the traditional hierarchy of evidence is most appropriate. In examples B, C and D below, different types of evidence will be stronger with regards to answering the literature review question:

Example B: When studies of patient or client experience are the best evidence

Imagine you are doing a literature review to explore patients' perceptions of their GP surgeries. Top of your hierarchy of evidence will be cross-sectional studies (surveys and questionnaires) and qualitative approaches. You would need to be aware that questionnaires will obtain a different type of data from that obtained by in-depth qualitative interviews.

For example B, the following evidence will be strongest in addressing this literature review question (strongest evidence first):

1 Systematic reviews of qualitative studies of patient perceptions
2 Quantitative and qualitative studies of patient perceptions
3 Expert opinion
4 Anecdotal opinion.

Example C: When observational studies are the best evidence
Imagine you are doing a literature review to explore whether students comply with handwashing procedures in clinical practice. In this case, top of your hierarchy will be research in which direct observation has been employed as the main method in the first instance. This is because indirect reports of handwashing practices, for example questionnaire/surveys, report what practitioners say they do rather than what they actually do. You would search for indirect reports of handwashing practice as a second line of evidence.

For example C, the following evidence will be strongest in addressing this literature review question (strongest evidence first):

1 Systematic reviews of observational studies
2 Observational studies
3 Expert opinion
4 Anecdotal opinion.

Once you have identified your own hierarchy of evidence, you are then advised to concentrate your initial searches for this type of evidence in the first instance. You should write up your rationale for doing this in the methods section of your literature review.

Should I always focus my search on research findings?

It has been suggested throughout this book that the type of literature you need to use to answer your research question depends on your question. This is probably the most important message of this entire book! However, it is also likely that primary research articles will comprise the main body of your literature review. As we have discussed before, this is because they are likely to provide the most relevant and best quality of evidence for answering your research question, which is likely to arise from your practice environment. However, where there is little research evidence, practice or anecdotal evidence can be used as evidence in your results, but it is important that you acknowledge that this is weaker evidence than research. It is important to remember that expert opinion remains 'opinion' only and is therefore not strong evidence. Indeed, it could be argued that some experts might become so engrossed in their subject that they are less able to provide an objective assessment of the topic area (Greenhalgh 1997). As a general rule, if the main body of your literature review does not focus on the findings of empirical research, make sure you can justify why this is the case.

The exception to this is where the research question for a literature review is only answerable through the use of theory, practice or policy literature.

Example D: When research is not relevant for your review
You are doing a literature review to explore how the media reports health and social care issues; for example, the scare over the swine influenza virus. To answer this question, the literature that will be most useful to you will be the media reports themselves. You are likely to write an introductory chapter on the background to this type of influenza, but your research question can only be answered by searching for and analysing media reports. In this case, you would not search for research in the first instance, as this would not help you to address the research question directly. Top of your hierarchy of evidence would be media reports.

For example D, the following evidence will be strongest in addressing this literature review question. In this case, there is really only media evidence that can answer your question but you might differentiate between different types of media.

1 Media reports of swine influenza virus. (You might divide your analysis between tabloid and broadsheet coverage of the swine influenza virus.)

In summary

You will encounter a wide variety of literature related to your question when you undertake your literature review. This is likely to include primary data from quantitative and/or qualitative studies and reviews of these studies, in addition to non-research papers (discussion papers, letters, and so on). Once you have identified your research question, you need to be specific about the evidence necessary to address your question. A summary of this information is included in this chapter to assist you in making sense of the literature you come across. The traditional concept of the hierarchy of evidence has been discussed but it is emphasized that the type of literature you need to address your research is entirely dependent on your research question, and that you should be guided by this to determine what literature you seek. This is referred to as developing your own hierarchy for addressing your literature review question. The next chapter examines the importance of identifying an appropriate searching strategy to find the literature you need.

Key points

- You are likely to encounter a wide range of information that is relevant to your literature review question.
- It is important to identify the types of information that you need to address your literature review question.
- Certain types of evidence will be essential for answering your literature review question. Other evidence will be less important.
- It is useful to develop your own *hierarchy of evidence* to determine what evidence is most relevant to your literature review question.
- You will use this hierarchy of evidence when you consider your search terms and inclusion criteria.

4

How do I search for literature?

Developing a systematic approach to searching for literature

Once you have established your research question and have identified the types of literature that will be most useful to you in addressing the research question, you need to develop a *systematic search strategy* that will enable you to identify and locate the most relevant range of published material in order to answer your research question in the most comprehensive way.

A literature review that is approached systematically is very different from one that is approached in a haphazard manner. A thorough and comprehensive search strategy will help to ensure that you identify key literature/texts on your topic and that you will find the relevant research that has been undertaken in your area. Without a thorough search strategy, your searching will be random and disorganized, and the reader of the review will not be confident that you have identified all the relevant research papers relating to your topic. When you undertake a comprehensive search strategy and document this, the reader of your review will be confident that you have been thorough in your search and that your findings are representative of the literature. This is essential to ensure that you identify as much of the literature that is relevant to your review as possible, within the time and financial restrictions of your review.

A systematic search strategy means that you identify which type of literature to look for to help address your review question. You develop search terms that are logical and relevant to your search and are derived from your literature review question. Using inclusion and exclusion criteria, you search for literature using your search terms through all the relevant databases. You then supplement this electronic search by hand searching the most frequently cited journals and looking through the reference list of the journal articles you find. This process gives you the greatest chance of identifying the maximum amount of literature so that you avoid either 'cherry-picking' the literature you want to include, or including just the first relevant literature that you come across. We discuss how you achieve a comprehensive search strategy in more detail in this chapter.

Components of a systematic search

Searching for literature is a two-stage approach:

- Stage 1: Plan your strategy
- Stage 2: Implement this strategy.

If emphasizing the role of planning, in addition to implementing your strategy, sounds a little obvious, then the reason for breaking it down into these two parts is that it draws attention to the importance of thinking carefully about your search before you begin. It is common for students to get to the end of their literature review and only then realize (or have someone else point out) that they have not searched for a critical keyword. Hence the conclusions for the literature review become far less reliable. You are less likely to find yourself in this situation if you plan your search strategy out in advance and discuss this with your supervisor. This is not to say that new ideas for **keywords** will not arise as you progress with your study and of course you should integrate these into your search strategy as they come up, but thinking through all the possible keywords and terms that cover every aspect of your research question is vital at an early planning stage.

Identifying what you need to search for

Once you have defined your research question, you should have an idea about your own *hierarchy of evidence*, as discussed in Chapter 3; that is, what type of evidence will best help you to answer your research question. Remember that you will normally be looking for primary research in the first instance. Whether you are looking for qualitative or quantitative research, and the type of qualitative or quantitative studies, will depend on your research question. In other words, your research question is the basis from which you can start to develop *your own hierarchy of evidence* that will answer your literature review question. Remember that your *hierarchy of evidence* is only a guide and be prepared to find relevant literature outside these guiding principles. Once you have worked out what you need to search for, you can begin to develop **inclusion and exclusion criteria** to guide your search.

Developing inclusion criteria based on your own hierarchy of evidence

Keeping focussed

If you identify clear and well-defined inclusion and exclusion criteria, this will ensure that you do not get sidetracked with data (literature) that are not strictly relevant to your review. Thus, setting appropriate criteria assists you in keeping your study focussed.

Inclusion and exclusion criteria help you to identify what you need to search for in your review. They enable the literature reviewer to identify the literature that addresses the research question and that which does not. The criteria you develop will be guided by the wording of your research question and your own hierarchy of evidence. Identifying inclusion and exclusion criteria will enable you to articulate the focus of your research and they will guide and focus your literature searching so that you do not go off track.

Examples

If you are looking to determine whether a new drug is effective or not, then finding out about patients' or clients' experiences of the drug will not help you to answer *your question*, although it will provide useful data and you might include this in the background information. What you need to find are studies reporting experiments (for example, randomized controlled trials) that have assessed the effectiveness of the drug.

To give another example, if you are interested in exploring students' experience of illicit drug use at university, you need to access only studies that report students' experience rather than related but more general literature that does not address your research question; for example, literature exploring the effect of a conviction for illicit drug use on future career prospects.

Thinking back to the examples given in Chapter 3, let's consider what some basic inclusion and exclusion criteria for these studies might be.

Example A

Imagine you are doing a literature review exploring the effectiveness of a particular treatment or care intervention. Let's say your review question is, *'How effective are anti-bullying policies in preventing bullying behaviour in school age children?'*

Inclusion criteria: Studies that explore the effectiveness of bullying policies.

Exclusion criteria: Studies that explore aspects other than the effectiveness of bullying policies.

Example B

Imagine you are doing a literature review to explore patients' perceptions of their GP surgeries.

Inclusion criteria: Surveys and questionnaires that explore patients' perceptions of the care received in GP practices.

Exclusion criteria: Studies that explore aspects other than patients' perceptions of the care received in GP practices.

Example C

Imagine you are doing a literature review to explore whether students comply with handwashing procedures in clinical practice.

Inclusion criteria: Observational studies of the ward environment.

Exclusion criteria: Studies that discuss or compare the effectiveness of different hand hygiene approaches.

Developing more detailed inclusion and exclusion criteria

Inclusion and exclusion criteria also allow you to demonstrate the scope and detail of your review that you would not be able to demonstrate in the review question itself. Therefore, when you are reading literature reviews, and when you are writing your own, the inclusion and exclusion criteria provide vital information about the scope and relevance of the review. It is on these criteria that your review and the reviews of others are judged for generalizability and relevance. For example, imagine your review is exploring the dietary intake of those who use illicit drugs. This is the title of your review and also forms the research question. However, this title and research question does not specify which type of drug users you are primarily interested in. This will be evident in the inclusion and exclusion criteria.

More detailed inclusion and exclusion criteria will help you to develop a strategy for searching for the literature that is directly related to your research question. Literature that is not relevant to you must be discarded in the first instance. You might return to this literature at a later stage but it should not be incorporated in the main body of the review if it does not directly address the research question. This is very important and you must resist the temptation to include interesting literature if it is not relevant, as it will detract from your review – however interesting it may seem! Once you have identified in general terms the type of literature you need, you can identify additional criteria that will help you refine your search strategy.

The inclusion and exclusion criteria will be specific to your individual literature review but examples of appropriate inclusion and exclusion criteria might be as follows.

Example of inclusion criteria:

- Primary research relating to nutrition and those who use heroin or cocaine
- English language only
- Published literature only
- 1995 onwards.

Example of exclusion criteria

- Primary research relating to those who use drugs other than heroin and cocaine
- Not English language
- Unpublished research
- Pre-1995.

The main rationales for setting your inclusion and exclusion criteria are:

- to provide clear information about the remit of your review; and
- to focus your literature search.

When thinking about your inclusion and exclusion criteria, think about the dates that are relevant for your review. If a pivotal event happened at a certain time that is relevant to your review, you might only be interested in literature published after that event. In this case, you set literature published after this date as one of your inclusion criteria. If you are only interested in local or national literature because you feel that your topic is mainly relevant to your own country, then you can state this in your inclusion criteria. Equally, if you are interested in international literature, you should state why this is the case. If you are mainly interested in a specific aspect of the main topic, then you should state this in your inclusion and exclusion criteria as well.

Practical reasons for setting inclusion and exclusion criteria

You are likely to find that some of your criteria are set for practical reasons, given that you will have a limited time frame within which to search and undertake your review. For example, you are likely to limit your search to more recent literature and to omit unpublished literature from your review. Neither of these restrictions is ideal and, under optimum conditions, you would obtain all available literature that is related to your topic. For example, there might be a seminal piece of work that is highly relevant to your review but which was published before the date limitations you set. Seminal work refers to work that has become key subject knowledge in the area, such as Einstein's theory of relativity. If you set time restrictions to your search for literature, you would miss this seminal document, although of course it might be referred to in other papers that you encounter.

Justifying your inclusion and exclusion criteria

In reality, your inclusion and exclusion criteria will be a combination of limits that are necessary to focus your search and pragmatic limitations that are required due to the resources available to you. The important point is that you are able to justify why you have set the inclusion and exclusion criteria, which should be determined by the needs of your review rather than your own convenience. For example, it would not be appropriate to include only those studies that you can access electronically if a hard-bound copy of an article you require is available in the local library. Therefore, when you write your inclusion and exclusion criteria, it is useful to justify them. So, for example, if your research question is exploring health and social care professionals' reaction to the Mental Capacity Act 2005, you would want to include only literature that was published after 2005. When you give your justification for the inclusion and exclusion criteria, you demonstrate to the reader that these criteria are carefully considered and fit the needs of the review.

Re-checking your inclusion and exclusion criteria

It is important to refer to and review your inclusion and exclusion criteria while you are searching. It is also important to keep checking that these criteria remain relevant to your research question – you may need to amend either or both of these as your literature review progresses. You need to make sure that you do not get sidetracked by interesting but peripheral issues if these are not directly related to your research question. However, if you encounter an interesting angle to the literature you are searching for and decide to change your research question so that this can be incorporated, then this could be appropriate. If you do this, you need to make sure that the whole literature review reflects the changes you have made.

> Your inclusion and exclusion criteria need to be stated clearly in your methods section when you write up your review.

Using databases to find evidence that fits with your inclusion criteria

Once you know what type of literature you need to address your research question and have developed your inclusion and exclusion criteria, you are ready to begin searching for literature. There are four main ways of searching for literature. These are electronic searching using computer-held databases, searching reference lists, hand searching relevant journals specific to the research topic and contacting authors directly. These four approaches will be considered in this and the following section.

Electronic searching

The main focus of your literature search is likely to be using online **subject-specific electronic databases** for which you have access through your academic library. Searching for literature when undertaking a literature review has been revolutionized in recent years by the advances in electronic databases. In years gone by, those reviewing the literature would have to search through hard-bound volumes of subject-indexed references in which previously published literature was categorized. Clearly, these volumes could not be immediately updated, as to do so required a reprint of the entire publication, which took place often on a yearly basis. Searching for literature has become a far easier and efficient process with the advent of electronic databases for literature searching.

Computerized databases are huge subject indexes of journal articles and other literature related to the topic for which you are searching. They operate along a similar principle to that of a non-academic search engine, such as Google, in which you enter a search term and are directed to relevant websites. However, academic search engines are far more specific than a general search engine, and they allow you to do advanced searching using different combinations of words and have direct access to academic journals and books. Therefore, they will only direct you to relevant academic literature, rather than the thousands of hits you get when you do a Google search. To search effectively, you need to identify appropriate keywords, which is discussed below. When you search using these keywords, in different combinations, you will be directed to references for journal articles or books that have the same keywords. Some databases give you direct access to the journal article itself. You might also be familiar with searching for academic references using Google Scholar. While this database can be a good place to start searching, especially in identifying key terms, it does not have access to as many academic journals as the more subject-specific databases and does not have an advanced search facility, which we discuss later in this chapter. Various databases will be available through the university or hospital library to which you belong. The first step is to identify databases to which you have access and to establish the relevance of these for your search strategy.

Commonly held databases

AMED: Allied health care including complementary medicine
ASSIA: Applied Social Sciences Indexes and Abstracts
Autism Data: Published research papers, books, articles and videos on autism
British Nursing Index: Nursing, midwifery and community health care
CAB Abstracts: Human nutrition, biotechnology, infectious diseases
Campbell Collaboration: Systematic reviews of the effects of social interventions
Cancer Library: National Cancer Institute, USA
CASonline: Provided by the British Institute of Learning Disabilities
CINAHL: Nursing and allied health care from North America and Europe
CIRRIE: Centre for International Rehabilitation Research Information
Cochrane Library: Systematic reviews of evidence-based health care
DARE: Database of Abstracts of Reviews of Effects
DUETs: Database of Uncertainties about the Effects of Treatments
HMIC: Non-clinical topics including inequalities in health and user involvement
Joanna Briggs Institute: Nursing-focussed systematic reviews
MEDLINE: Extensive medical and nursing database
OTdirect: OT specific study notes, practice updates and training listings

OTseeker: Abstracts of systematic reviews and RCTs relevant to occupational therapy

PEDRO: Physiotherapy evidence database

Planex: Local public policy and governance including social work

PsychINFO: Psychology, psychiatry, child development, psychological care

PubMed: Medical and health professions

NARIC (National Rehabilitation Information Center): Disability and rehabilitation

NHS Clinical Knowledge Summaries: Evidence-based information on common conditions managed in primary care

Rehabdata: Disability and rehabilitation

Social Care Online: Social and community care

Social Services Abstracts: Abstracts from journal articles on social work, welfare and policy

Sociological Abstracts: Sociology and political theory

Source: Management and practice of primary health care and disability in developing countries

TRIP database: Evidence-based medicine and healthcare resources on the web

Web of Science: Includes Science Citation Index and Social Sciences Citation Index

ZETOC: British Library's electronic table of contents

For those undertaking a nursing-based literature review, CINAHL would be an appropriate start. CINAHL covers a wide range of international nursing literature, which commenced in 1982. There are various different search strategies that include, for example, the possibility to search for research articles only. For those undertaking social work-based studies, Social Care Online is a good place to start. Medline is a more generic database, offering reference to medical, nursing and social care literature. It is important to note that while Medline is a huge database, it contains references to journal articles only, whereas other databases such as CINAHL reference a wider range of book and non-research information, in addition to journal articles. In principle, all those undertaking a review of the literature are strongly recommended to consult with the academic subject librarian at their university for further advice concerning the appropriate use of databases for a particular study.

If your library runs a session on using databases make sure you attend, as this will assist you to make the most of your searching sessions. Remember that the processes of using the databases will vary from one to another and they will be updated regularly.

The main thing to emphasize with electronic searching is that it is a skill that you need to practise on a regular basis. Make use of the training sessions offered in your academic library. You will not complete your search in half a day; in fact, if you are a novice researcher, it is only by the time that you finish your literature review that you are likely to feel really competent in using the search engines. When you change to a new database, you need to learn about how the new database operates.

Getting started

Start by selecting the database you are going to use. You will need to justify in your review which databases you selected and why. All databases operate slightly differently and it takes time and skill to learn how to use them effectively. However, the following principles apply.

Identifying keywords

In the first instance, you should identify the **keywords** that capture the essence of the topic or question for the review. The reason behind identifying keywords is that when journal articles are indexed and entered onto a database, they are indexed using keywords. You need to enter these same keywords to retrieve these articles. Refer back to your inclusion and exclusion criteria and check that you have incorporated the key concepts within these criteria in your key terms.

Thinking of all the keywords relevant to your literature review question is essential if you are going to identify a comprehensive range of literature.

Brainstorm as many keywords as you can think of that represent your review question. Remember that the topic or question might be categorized in different ways by different researchers. Therefore, you should think of as many different words that describe your topic and be as creative as possible at this stage. Think of synonyms, words that mean the same thing, and have both words in your selection of keywords. Think of phrases or terms that are no longer used and include these in your keywords. Now is not the time for political correctness! This is because relevant articles might be indexed under a term that is no longer used. For example, if your area uses the term 'learning difficulty', include this term as a keyword, but also include the term 'learning disability' in case there is literature that is indexed under one term and not the other. It is also useful to use a thesaurus to identify alternative words. You need to consider whether there are different meanings to the keywords that you identify in different countries, especially given that databases have different biases. For example, CINAHL has a strong North American bias, and the BNI has a British focus. It is also wise to remember that you may identify new keywords as you progress with your search and encounter alternative ways in which your research topic is represented in the literature. You will find that you identify new possible search terms as your search progresses. For example, say that you are searching for literature on a new technique in the rehabilitation of a patient following knee injury. You can search for the names of the procedure but remember that the rehabilitation procedure might be referred to in many different ways that might come to light once you begin searching.

How many searches you make will depend on your research question and the variety of terms used in relation to this topic. You might need to break down the topic into smaller units. For example, if you are researching the use of illicit drugs, your keywords might include: illicit drugs, illegal drugs and drug abuse. Then you might break down the topic by searching on individual illicit drugs: heroin, cocaine, and so on.

Using the specific database searching facilities

In addition to identifying keywords, most databases have the * or $ facility that enables you to identify all possible endings of the key term you write. For example nurs* or nurs$ will identify articles containing nurse, nursing, nurses, and so on. Therefore, using this instruction will ensure you access all possible endings of the main term you have selected. Then, when you have identified all your keywords, consider how many of these have endings that you can truncate and this will make your search easier. You are advised to ensure that you are familiar with the instructions for shortening key terms for each database you use.

Using the Thesaurus/MeSH headings within a database

In addition to identifying your own keywords, many of the databases have developed their own keywords for popular search terms and have used these to index literature. These can be regarded as 'controlled' key terms and those which have been used by the database to index papers. If you use the Thesaurus/**MeSH** (Medical Subject Headings) you are likely to get a reduced number of hits, as you will not access the whole scope of papers. This can be useful if you are inundated with results from your search but remember to consider whether you are omitting relevant papers if you edit your search using 'controlled' keywords only rather than your own keywords. It can be useful to demonstrate a comparison of the results that you get using your own keywords and the 'controlled' keywords within a database thesaurus.

Using Boolean operators

Once you have made a list of your keywords for each aspect of your topic, you are ready to start searching. It is advisable to start your search at the *advanced searching* option of the database rather than to under-take a *basic search,* as the basic search is very limited and is likely to yield very many hits that you will not be able to make sense of. When you enter the advanced searching option of the database, you are likely to find a box to enter your first keyword and then other boxes to enter alternative keywords. This is where you will be able to make use of the AND/OR/NOT commands. These commands use the principles of Boolean logic and are an essential feature of all databases. Make sure you are familiar with these commands.

- AND searches for both terms and hence limits the search.
- OR searches for either term and hence widens the search.
- NOT excludes the term from a search. Many experts recommend caution when using the NOT command in case you omit potentially relevant papers.

Let's say you are looking for literature on childhood obesity. If your keywords include 'child' AND 'eating disorder' AND 'nutrition', your search will be limited to literature that contains *all* keywords in either the title, **abstract** or whole paper (depending on your selection as discussed below).

Once you are happy with the keywords or abbreviations you have set up, you can start your search, searching the databases using *all the different combinations of keywords* that you have, using the AND/OR/ NOT commands as appropriate. For example, if you are searching for literature on nutritional status of drug users, you will identify as many keywords as you can for both nutritional status and drug users and then search the database combining the keywords you have:

> Illicit drug use AND diet$
> Illicit drug use AND nutrition$
> Illegal drug use AND diet$

And so on.

It is also possible to combine the above two searches using the OR command:

> Illicit drug use AND diet$ OR nutrition$

If you want to exclude heroin users, you can use the NOT command so that literature relating to heroin will not be identified:

> Illegal drug use AND diet$ NOT heroin

Setting limitations on your search

You can make various specifications about refining your search. For example, you can specify whether you would like to search for your keyword throughout the whole article, or whether you are going to limit your search to the **abstract** or **title**. Clearly, if you limit your search to the identification of the term in just the title, you will exclude a lot of references that might be relevant to you, even though the title does not use the key terms you have identified. Conversely, if you search through every article for your keyword, you are likely to be overwhelmed with literature. Depending on your topic, you are probably best to limit your search to the title and abstract; however, if your topic is hard to identify, and your keywords not often indexed in the title or abstract, then you might need to search through the whole paper for your keyword. It is also possible to limit your search by date or type of paper – you might want to restrict your search to **research papers** in the first instance.

What to do if you have too many hits

If you have too many hits – let's say in the thousands – you cannot simply ignore them and select just a few that seem to address your literature review question. To do this would be to ignore papers that are relevant to you and to cherry pick the literature you include. This way, you are likely to bias your findings. Instead, consider why you have too many hits. Are your search terms too broad? Is your question focussed enough? It is preferable to re-consider your question for your literature review and to focus the question so that it leads you to a narrower range of literature.

Keeping a record of your search

Remember to record and document all the details of your searches including keywords and databases searched. This is needed for your own records – one search will quickly merge into another if you do not record what you have done. It is also needed when you write up your literature review, as you need to demonstrate that your search was thorough and systematic.

You are likely to find that you develop new ideas for the search terms you use as you start the search process. You need to keep a clear audit trail of this. Without clear documentation, you will not remember what you have searched for and what you have not yet searched for. You might find, for example, a key theme is called by a different name or phrase that you had not previously thought of. Be aware of this and be prepared to search using new and different terms – keeping a record at all times. If you do not have any 'hits' from your search, then record this but keep searching with different keywords until you identify literature that is linked to your topic area.

Using different databases

Once you have identified the key literature on your topic using one database, it is important to repeat the search using another database. If you find that the same references are thrown up, then you can be confident that your strategy is well focussed and that you are accessing the relevant literature on your topic.

When to stop searching

When you find that you are getting the same references from different database searches, you might feel it is appropriate to scale down your search. Discuss this with your supervisor. If new references are constantly being thrown up, you will need to continue searching until later searches reveal little or no new information. This is where the importance of having a research question that is neither too big nor too small is evident. Ideally at undergraduate level, you will retrieve 10–20 references that are well focussed on your topic; you may have more for a postgraduate study. As mentioned previously, it would be difficult to address your research question with fewer references but you would be inundated with literature if many more references were identified.

Formal recording of your search results from electronic searches

You need to record your search strategy formally in your final presentation of your literature review. For example, if you are searching for primary research articles concerned with childhood obesity and mental health, you might initially undertake two basic searches and then combine these searches:

Database: CINAHL 1994 – **Search term:** child*/$
Total number of hits: 30,0000

Database: CINAHL 1994 – **Search term:** obesity (no truncation)
Total number of hits: 15,0000

Database: CINAHL 1994 – **Search term:** mental health (no truncation)
Total number of hits: 30,0000

Database: CINAHL 1994 – **Search terms:** child*$ AND obesity AND mental health
Total number of hits: 35

You can then document the other searches you undertook in this manner and demonstrate how you combined these searches with others in order to obtain the most relevant hits. It is important that you demonstrate the success of your search strategy and how many hits each search yielded.

Limitations of an electronic search

It should be emphasized that, despite the advances in electronic searching, computerized searching tools are not 100 per cent comprehensive and will not identify all the relevant literature on your topic. This has been well documented (Wong *et al.* 2004; McKibbon *et al.* 2006; Wilczynski *et al.* 2007; Papaioannou *et al.* 2010). The reason for this is that some relevant literature might have been categorized using different keywords and therefore would not be identified by one particular search strategy. Or, if you are searching for a hard to reach topic, you might find that the topic is not indexed in literature in which it is included. This means that a database search will not pick up this relevant literature, making it very difficult for you to complete your search. Although using various keywords will help you identify literature that is not identified on the first search, it is still possible for literature to remain unidentified even though it is highly relevant to addressing the research question.

Additional search strategies

The consensus of expert opinion (Wong *et al.* 2004; McKibbon *et al.* 2006; Wilczynski *et al.* 2007; Papaioannou *et al.* 2010) is that using carefully developed keywords will maximize the success of your search strategy. However, even a carefully executed electronic search strategy will need to be supplemented using additional search methods. This conclusion has been reached by researchers who have cross-referenced the results of electronic searching with literature found in a more 'ad hoc' way and found that, for various reasons, relevant pieces of research were omitted from the results of electronic searches. For example, Betrán *et al.* (2005) found that 20 per cent of studies in their review were not identified through a database search. Mattioli *et al.* (2012) found that although good search terms made the database search more accurate, supplementary search methods identified more literature.

Electronic searches are likely to be the main component of your search strategy, but they should not be the only component. It is important to remember that there is no single strategy that will ensure that you retrieve all the information you need to address your research question. Further strategies, including reference list searching, hand searching through reference lists and author searching, will add to the thoroughness of your search strategy.

Greenhalgh and Peacock (2005) emphasize the importance of using many approaches to identifying appropriate literature when undertaking a literature search and argue that systematic reviewers cannot rely on computerized databases to yield all the information they need for their study. It may seem haphazard to employ a variety of methods to search for literature, especially if these appear somewhat random, such as scrutinizing recent copies of particular journals. However, given the limitations of using electronic searching alone, the wider search strategy, as long as it is organized and its relevance is justified in the remit of the study, can be part of a comprehensive systematic approach. Greenhalgh and Peacock (2005) refer to this process as **snowball sampling** – where the sampling strategy develops according to the requirements of the study and is responsive to the literature already obtained. For example, if useful articles are found in a particular journal, then this journal is further scrutinized for other relevant material. This strategy cannot be pre-specified and is dependent on the results of early literature searching. Greenhalgh and Peacock (2005) reported 'snowball sampling' to be the most effective approach to literature searching in their systematic review.

> The point to remember is that these additional search strategies are not 'haphazard' if they are combined with an electronic search. Using additional strategies only would be haphazard if they were the *only* means of searching for literature.

RSS feeds (Rich Site Summary or Really Simple Syndication)

RSS feeds are automated links that you can set up from blogs, news websites, journals which can alert you to newly published articles and other information on your literature review topic. RSS feeds will assist you by giving the most up-to-date information and ideas related to your topic or literature review question and are likely to be additional to those you would access through an academic search engine. Critical appraisal of the information sourced through these sites is important and will be discussed in Chapter 5; however, using RSS feeds will give you access to new ideas and information as they are generated within your field. These are useful to consider even if they do not lead to a useful contribution to your project.

Searching the reference lists

Once you have identified the key articles that relate to your research question, it is useful to scrutinize the reference lists of those key articles for further references that may be useful to you.

Hand searching relevant journals

If you have been able to identify that many of your key articles that are relevant to your research question are located in one or two journals, it might be useful to you to hand search these journals to see whether you can identify other relevant articles that have not been identified through other search strategies. Searching through the contents pages of these journals may identify other relevant material.

Author searching

The same principle applies to author searching. If you find that many of your key articles are by the same author(s), then it may be useful to carry out an author search in order to identify whether the author(s) have published other work that has not been identified in the electronic search. This might also lead you towards work in progress.

A combination of these strategies will ensure that you have the most comprehensive search strategy and therefore the most chance of retrieving the information that is relevant to your research question. However, you can never be certain that you have obtained all the literature on a particular topic. For this reason, it is recommended that you avoid statements that declare there is no literature on a particular topic and state instead that no literature was *identified* on the topic in question.

Locating unpublished literature

There is concern about including only literature that has been published. This is because of the risk of publication bias; that is, journals tend to publish research that shows the positive effect of an intervention rather than a negative effect or no effect. This is likely to be particularly true of pharmaceutical studies where, it is sometimes claimed, only the studies which show a positive effect are published (Goldacre 2012). Hence, only including published literature could bias your review. There might be a lot of 'hidden' evidence about your topic that remains unpublished because the results showed no effect. This literature is often referred to as 'grey' literature and refers to literature that is not published or generally in the public domain, such as a dissertation. Non-academic journals might also be referred to as grey literature and other information such as hospital policies also fall into this category. As a novice researcher you would not be expected to access 'grey' literature that is difficult to find. Unpublished literature can be hard to identify or get hold of. Searching for unpublished, or grey, literature will usually be beyond the scope of the literature reviewer at undergraduate level, as he or she is unlikely to have the time and resources to search for unpublished research. However, it is important to acknowledge this when you discuss the limitations of your review methodology.

Recording your search results from additional methods of searching

You should document the results of your additional methods of searching in the same way as your database searches.

Checking the abstracts of your search against the inclusion criteria

Once you have undertaken a thorough search, you are ready to combine the results of all your electronic and additional searches and compare the abstracts from the papers you have identified with your inclusion criteria. The abstract of a paper is a short summary of the content of the paper, and usually includes the aims, methods, results and discussion if the paper is a research paper. Most databases will provide the abstract of the papers they index. Some databases will also provide a link to the full paper but you do not need this at this stage.

So, to get started, with the inclusion criteria in one hand and the abstracts in the other (so to speak), work through each abstract and accept those that meet your inclusion criteria and reject those that do not. If you cannot tell from the abstract, it is advisable to access the full copy of the paper in order to do this. By undertaking this process, you should be able to edit your list of 'hits' to those papers that are directly relevant to your research question.

If you were undertaking a detailed systematic review, in order to enhance the rigour of this process you could have a colleague work on the same set of abstracts and, once you had both completed the process of accepting and rejecting abstracts, you could compare your results. This process is possible even at undergraduate level if you pair up with a colleague who is doing a literature review and ask him or her to undertake this process alongside you and then return the favour. Remember to write this up when you write up how you undertook your literature review.

When you have reached a conclusion about which literature meets your inclusion criteria, have a closer look at each abstract that you have. Consider whether you have identified the literature that is highest in your own *hierarchy of evidence* for answering your research question. If you are searching for articles of primary research of a particular type but are failing to identify these, you need to document this. This enables the reader to develop a sense of the ease with which you were able to identify literature and the outcome of your searches.

Document the process of identifying literature from your inclusion criteria for your review

You need to document the process of refining down your search so that the reader is satisfied that relevant papers have not been omitted on the way. The following flow chart is adapted from the PRISMA diagram, which has been developed to help authors of systematic reviews report their studies in a complete and transparent way (http://www.prisma-statement.org/statement.htm):

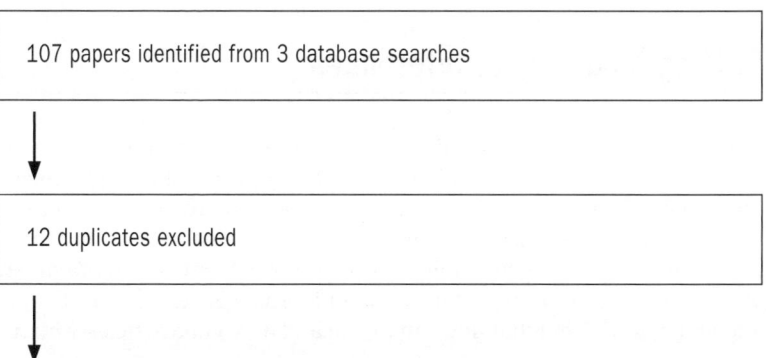

107 papers identified from 3 database searches

12 duplicates excluded

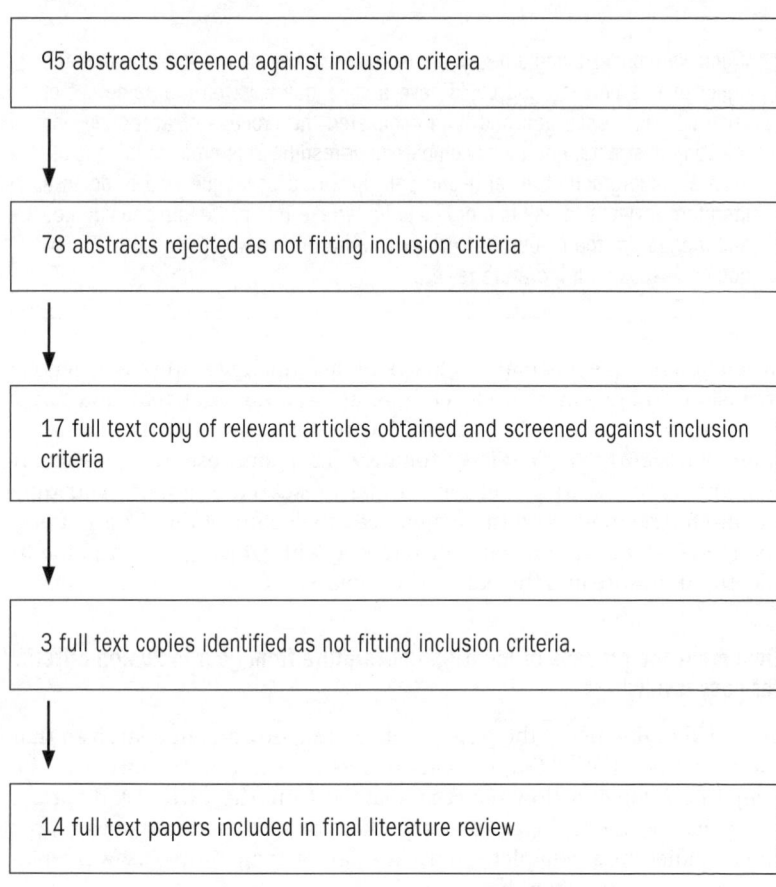

95 abstracts screened against inclusion criteria

78 abstracts rejected as not fitting inclusion criteria

17 full text copy of relevant articles obtained and screened against inclusion criteria

3 full text copies identified as not fitting inclusion criteria.

14 full text papers included in final literature review

Getting hold of your references

Once you have a list or a pile of abstracts that meet your inclusion criteria, the next step is to obtain the paper copies of these references. The references to which you are directed are likely to be found in journals, books and other publications. Your academic subject librarian will be able to help you locate publications with which you are not familiar. Most university libraries will have many journals accessible electronically and you will find that you can locate and download articles without leaving your computer. The online journals will be available from your library website but will be at different databases from those accessed to identify the literature. You are strongly advised to familiarize yourself with the journals to which you have easy access through your library. If the reference you require is not available electronically, then you will need to access the bound volumes that are available as hard copies in the library. If the references that are vital to your research question are not available electronically or in bound volumes in your local library, then you will either need to arrange to visit another library or arrange an inter-library loan. It is important to remember that obtaining these references can be expensive and time-consuming, so you will need to make a decision about the effort you are going to put in to access the references you need. For those references that are of interest to but not crucial to your research question, and which are not easily available, it is reasonable to explain in your methodology that the retrieval of these articles was not possible due to the time and financial limitations of the study. However, you will be given credit for the effort you make in obtaining key references for your literature review.

Managing your references

There are many ways to manage your references. It does not matter which way you select, as long as you manage them. Whether you record your references on a computer or on paper, it is vitally important to back up all your records and keep them in a safe place from the moment that you begin the search process. There are three main choices for managing your references:

1 Keeping a hard, paper copy
2 Keeping an electronic copy/PDF on your computer
3 Using a reference manager software such as *Endnote, Reference manager*, or *Ref works.*

If you are keeping records on a computer, remember to have a back-up copy at all times. Keep all of your records up to date. If you are using an electronic reference manager, you are advised to attend a training course before you begin so that you learn how to get the most out of your software. Whichever way you manage your references, it is important to re-emphasize that you need to keep track of your references. Write them down in full every time you read something useful. It is very frustrating to have to track down page numbers or editions at the last minute just because you used something in the write-up that you had not anticipated including.

Strengths and limitations of your search strategy

Clearly, those doing a more detailed systematic review would make every effort to retrieve the articles relevant to their study. Overall, you will be given credit for the effort you make in locating all the references that are central to your study; however, you will not be unduly penalized if you cannot get hold of hard-to-reach articles that are not critical in answering your research question. You should, however, write this up in your methodology section as a potential limitation of your study.

Another limitation of undertaking a literature review for the novice researcher is also apparent at this point. If you were undertaking a more detailed systematic review, it would be usual for a team of researchers to review each of the identified references and review its relevance for the literature review. The novice researcher is disadvantaged because these resources are unlikely to be available to them. This should also be discussed in the methods section of the literature review.

It should also be emphasized that you should never be tempted to use sources in your literature review if you have not read the source in its original form. If an interesting reference is referred to in another research paper, but the reference is hard to access, you should never attempt to incorporate this material into your review. It is better to cite the reference and explain that you were unable to obtain it than to pretend that you have. This is because without reading the original document, you are unable to critique the material (as described in the following chapter) and are likely to misrepresent the material. If you use secondary sources, the entire foundation for your literature review is challenged, as the point of undertaking a review is that you pull together the available literature and critique it for relevance to your research question. The use of secondary sources was discussed earlier and you are advised to avoid using them wherever possible.

Tips for writing up your search strategy

1 Remember that the aim of this section is to demonstrate how you undertook a systematic approach to your searching.
2 Discuss the approach you took to develop effective search strategies.
3 Keep a record of all the search terms used so that you can provide evidence of your approach.
4 Keep a record of the other approaches you employed to search for literature.
5 If you are inundated with hits, consider why this is and revise your question or your search terms. Do not include the 'first ten papers' or 'cherry pick' papers.
5 Be able to comment on the effectiveness of the approaches you used. For example, if electronic searching did not yield as many hits as you had hoped, discuss why this might have been.
6 Make every effort to obtain relevant literature.
7 It is more accurate to write 'I did not find any literature on X' rather than state categorically 'There is no literature on X'.

In summary

You should now be well aware of the importance of a systematic search strategy. This will ensure that you access a comprehensive range of literature that is relevant to your literature review question. The use of inclusion and exclusion criteria is also vital to ensure that the literature identified is relevant to your review question. The need to combine the electronic searching of relevant databases with additional strategies such as hand searching journals and reference lists has been discussed. You need to be aware that electronic searching can never be fully comprehensive and that 'snowball sampling', using many different strategies to identify literature, will usually be the most effective way of achieving the most comprehensive literature search. At the end of the search process, you will achieve a list of references that are relevant to your research question for your literature review, which you will be able to locate in your academic library. You will be given credit for the amount of effort you make in accessing these references.

At this point, you should be confident that you have identified the most relevant literature that will enable you to answer your research question. You should be aware of the strengths and limitations of your search strategy. It is now time to stand back and take a critical look at the literature you have identified. Ideally, you will have identified between 10 and 20 references that are key to your research question. If you have many more than this or far fewer you may consider altering the focus of your review so that the literature you have identified fits your research question rather than vice versa. This is a luxury that you have if you are undertaking your literature review as part of an academic degree and that you would not have with more formally commissioned research. The main point to remember is that your literature should address your research question. While theoretically you could write up a study that yielded no results, you will find it easier – and more interesting – to write up a study that did yield some information. If you do not have sufficient information to address your research question, you are advised to alter your question so that you can address it using the literature that you have identified.

Key points

- Before you start searching, you should identify the types of literature that will enable you to answer your research question (as discussed in Chapter 3).
- Your inclusion and exclusion criteria will be specific to your literature review.
- Your key search terms will be developed according to your inclusion criteria.
- Electronic databases will form the basis for your search.
- Your search will also include a variety of additional approaches including hand searching and reference list searching, RSS feeds, and so on.
- Keep a record of all your searching – most databases will allow you to save the search electronically.
- Keep a handwritten record of all additional searches too.

5

How do I critically appraise the literature?

- *Getting to know your literature*
- *Getting started with critical appraisal*
- *Be critical but not too critical!*
- *Do I need to critically appraise all the papers I refer to in my literature review?*
- *Critical appraisal tools*
- *Re-emphasizing the importance of getting to know your literature*
- *Undertaking critical appraisal of your papers for your review*
- *Critical appraisal of research*
- *How do I critique systematic reviews or good quality literature reviews?*
- *Critical appraisal tools for reviews or good quality literature reviews*
- *How do I critique quantitative studies?*
- *Critical appraisal tools for quantitative studies*
- *How do I critique qualitative studies?*
- *Critical appraisal of qualitative studies*
- *Critical appraisal tools for qualitative studies*
- *How do I critique theory?*

- *How do I critique practice literature?*
- *How do I appraise policy and guidelines?*
- *How do I appraise information on websites?*
- *What next, now that I have critically appraised all my literature?*
- *Tips for doing your critique of the literature*
- *In summary*
- *Key points*

Getting to know your literature

At this stage, you should have completed a comprehensive search for the literature relating to your review question, worked through each abstract to identify relevant papers and obtained the hard copies of these papers.

Think back to the structure of the literature review, for which you are likely to have:

- a literature review question (or research question) set in context within an introductory chapter including background literature
- a methods section incorporating your search strategy, method of appraisal and analysis of the literature
- presentation of your results/themes incorporating critical appraisal of the studies included
- discussion of your results and recommendations for practice.

The papers you have identified through your search relate specifically to your literature review question and will form the main body of 'results' or 'themes' for your review. Resist the temptation to refer to these findings in your introduction to your literature review. As these papers enable you to answer your research question, you do not want to hint at the answer in your introduction.

The next step is to work through these papers and identify what they tell you about your research question. This is the first stage of the data analysis process. You need to get to know the literature thoroughly so that you can determine whether it is really relevant to your review and to assess the quality of the literature to determine how much weight it should have in addressing your review question.

Read and re-read your papers

The first step is to *read* and *re-read* the papers you have so that you become familiar with their content.

It is important to get to know your literature in as much detail as possible. By going through each piece of literature, you will be able to confirm that it is relevant to your review. Even if you have followed your inclusion and exclusion criteria closely when identifying papers for your review, it is only when you come to read the papers thoroughly that you will be able to work out how relevant they are for answering your research question. For example, at first glance, a research paper might appear to address your research question directly; however, on closer inspection you might realize that the scope of the paper is very different from what your initial assessment had led you to believe and in fact has only indirect relevance to your research question.

At this stage, you are likely to revise your initial assessment of papers and may find that some that you thought were 'results' or 'findings' actually do not shed light on your research question. In this case, remove this paper from your pile of results and consider using them in your background or discussion chapter. Literature that supports the development of your research question is likely to go in your introduction and that which helps to explain findings is more likely to go in the discussion.

What literature do I have and how relevant is it?

Refer back to your inclusion criteria and hierarchy of evidence and consider the type of evidence you have. Identify what is a research paper, theory paper, guidelines, practice or discussion or other information. Refer back to the classification system described in Chapter 3 (Wallace and Wray 2006) and see if you can classify the literature you have. You will know by now the type of literature you are looking to include in your review and it is important to recognize when you have it. It will not always be clear whether the literature you have identified is theoretical, research, practice or policy and you might need to discuss this with your supervisor.

Depending on your literature review question, you are likely to have predominantly research papers, and you may have a combination of qualitative and quantitative research, maybe some systematic reviews but also other non-research information. Group your literature together so that you have all the qualitative research papers in one pile, the quantitative papers in another, and so on. When you have done this, you will be able to identify the types of literature you have for critical review.

It is quite normal to feel overwhelmed by the different types and quantity of literature you may have but if you follow a methodological process, you will be able to make sense of your literature

Have I identified literature at the top of my own hierarchy of evidence?

The question *'Have I identified literature at the top of my hierarchy of evidence?'* is important because, as we have seen, different types of evidence are required to answer different questions. It is useful at this point to work out whether you have identified your top priority literature required for answering your question. For example, if you are looking to find out if an intervention is effective or not but have not identified any randomized controlled trials (RCTs) in your search, then you cannot answer the question as well as you would have liked, or at least not with the precision you would have liked. Alternatively, if you are looking at young people's experience of foster care, but found no phenomenological studies exploring the experience of care, you might conclude that you do not have the ideal literature to address your question. To do this, refer back to your own hierarchy of evidence – the evidence you need to answer *your* research question. Remind yourself of exactly what type of literature you were looking for and decide how much of this top-level evidence – literature at the top of your hierarchy – you found. To do this, you need to study carefully the research methods used in each research paper that you have, in order to see if the methods used are those you were seeking. If you do not find the type of literature at the top of your hierarchy, keep on going as you may be able to address the question with other literature, as long as you identify in your methods section that your ideal literature of choice was not available. We discuss this later in the chapter.

What are the main findings/conclusions in my papers?

You need to be familiar with all the papers before you can move on to more detailed critical appraisal. If you have research papers, make sure you can describe what the research method was and what the main findings were. If you have quantitative research that includes statistics – and these seem daunting – then ignore the statistics in the first instance and concentrate on the way the findings are described. Ask yourself what similarities and differences there are in the data described. Then look to see whether the authors report these findings as 'significant', which means 'unlikely to have occurred by chance'. Quantitative results which are described as 'statistically significant' will carry more weight than those which are not. We discuss more detailed critical appraisal of each papers later in this chapter but at this stage it is important to get a feel for what each paper is telling you in broad terms. The important thing is that you can explain each paper in 'lay' language so that you are sure that you have a good general understanding of the findings and conclusions of each of the papers. It is always a good test of how well you know the literature if you can discuss the literature you have found in detail with your research supervisor without reference to the papers themselves or at least with minimal reference.

What are the strengths and weaknesses of this literature?

By asking the question *'What are the strengths and weaknesses of this literature?'* you will determine the quality of the literature you have and whether it is of high enough quality to include in your review and, if so, what weight it should have in answering your question. This process is generally referred to as 'critical appraisal'. Critical appraisal is not an exact science and you will need to make some judgement calls here. For example, if you have literature that is very relevant to your review, is *top of your hierarchy of evidence,* but does not appear to have been undertaken in a thorough manner, you need to consider this when you write up your review. Alternatively, you might have literature that seems to have been conducted in a very thorough manner, but which is less relevant to your question. If overall you do not have a lot of relevant literature, you might find that you include this literature. We will discuss this further later in the chapter.

Critical appraisal of the literature is the process of addressing each of the three questions posed above. The first two questions are fairly easily dealt with. It is the third question that will take you the most time and consideration. When you appraise the literature, you assess the quality of each individual piece of literature you have identified in order to determine how much weight it should have in your review. Some researchers have strict criteria on the quality of study they include in their review and if the study does not match up in terms of rigour of methods used, then this study will be excluded from the review. We discuss this later in the chapter. Suffice it to say, that as a novice researcher, you are advised to include everything that is relevant to your review (assuming that you are not inundated with literature), but should acknowledge the limitations of the literature and hence the weight or impact that the literature has in addressing your research question.

Getting started with critical appraisal

Critical appraisal is the structured assessment of the strengths and weaknesses of each paper to enable you to make an assessment as to the relevance of the paper to your own literature review question. In principle, all the published material you use as findings or results in your literature review should be critiqued for relevance and for its strengths and limitations. When you are analysing your results, you should avoid citing an author without some analysis or appraisal of the contribution this author makes to the development of your findings. Critical appraisal is therefore very important when you are discussing your results or findings. You do not need to demonstrate the same level of critical appraisal when you are summarizing well-known arguments at the beginning of your literature review, or summarizing arguments in your discussion.

The importance of critical appraisal

Let us refer back to Wakefield and his colleagues who published a paper in *The Lancet* in 1998, which caused so much concern and controversy; the authors have subsequently withdrawn the paper. The controversy surrounding the MMR vaccination is discussed elsewhere in relation to critical appraisal (Aveyard and Sharp 2013) but it is hard to find a better example, as the impact of the controversy is ongoing some 15 years later (Kmietowicz 2012; Wise 2013).

The MMR controversy

In this paper, Wakefield *et al.* described how they investigated a case series of 12 children who had been referred to their paediatric gastro-enterology unit with a history of normal development followed by loss of acquired skills including language, as well as suffering from diarrhoea and abdominal pains. The parents reported that the onset of symptoms was associated with the administration of the MMR vaccination in 8 of the 12 children and with measles infection in another child. Wakefield and colleagues concluded that the potential link between autism and bowel disease with the MMR vaccination should be investigated.

This paper caused huge concern among the general public and the possibility of a link between the MMR vaccination, autism and bowel disease was speculated upon in the media. The importance of critical appraisal of this paper cannot be over-emphasized. If you think back to the discussion about hierarchies of evidence discussed earlier, this evidence would probably be ranked as very weak evidence, whichever hierarchy you referred to, given the size of the sample and lack of a comparison group. You would probably therefore conclude that the evidence for a link between the MMR vaccination and autism/bowel disease is weak and you would not consider acting on this weak evidence in your clinical practice. Yet, it is unfortunate that such critical appraisal did not halt the media scare that ensued, which resulted in many parents not presenting their children for vaccination and in the vaccination rate dropping dangerously low. As a result of this scare, many further studies were undertaken and no further evidence has been found to substantiate Wakefield's claims. Finally, these studies were incorporated into a systematic review that again found no evidence of a link between the MMR vaccination and autism/bowel disease.

The MMR controversy illustrates the importance of critical appraisal of research and other information so that you can identify how strong and relevant the evidence is relating to a particular topic. In any literature review on the safety of MMR, this paper would not be presented as strong evidence.

Be critical but not too critical!

Those new to academic writing often fall into one of two categories. The first accept any piece of research or other information at face value and so accept what is written without question. They cite a reference without any statement about the quality or authenticity of the report. In writing a literature review, this is not appropriate because it is essential to analyse the quality of the information in order to determine the contribution of the information to the overall argument. Those new to academic discussion may perceive a paper that is published in a reputable journal to be above critique and so do not attempt any structured appraisal of the paper. Even a paper that is published in a reputable journal must be examined for the relevance that it demonstrates to the topic area. The second group interpret the term 'critical appraisal' to mean that they must criticize and find fault with everything that they read. They feel that unless they demonstrably 'tear to pieces' what they find, then they have not done their job. While it is possible to find faults with every piece of research, it needs to be remembered that no research is perfect. If only perfect research was included in a literature review, there would be no reviews at all!

Critical appraisal is one of the most important features of a literature review that distinguishes the review from a more traditional **essay**. Those undertaking a literature review should resist the temptation merely to make a statement and then to provide a reference that apparently reinforces this statement. If no other information is given about the reference that allegedly makes this assertion, the reader has no evidence that this reference is used appropriately.

To give a poor, hypothetical example: '*Smith (2013) argues that university students prefer lectures to tutorials*'. If this is the only information that is given, the reader is unaware of the context from which the author is writing. It is unclear whether the author is merely citing an opinion or referring to published research, or whether the paper is actually the report of empirical findings about students' learning preferences. Further information needs to be given.

To give another hypothetical example: '*In a questionnaire survey of 2000 students in London, Smith (2013) identified that 70 per cent of university students preferred . . .*'. You would then go on to include the strengths and limitations of this survey. For example, you would need to state that only 20 per cent of students responded and of those who did respond, many of them did not fully complete the questionnaire. You may then conclude that the data suggesting that 70 per cent of students preferred a certain learning style do not constitute very strong evidence. Alternatively, if the article by Smith (2013) is actually an account of the author's own preference at university, you might then articulate this as follows: '*Smith (2013) argues that from his own experience as a student in London, there was a strong feeling among his peer group that lectures were preferable to seminars*'. You then make it clear that Smith is not referring to a piece of empirical research but to his own experience. Having identified the context of Smith's argument, you then need to explore the relevance of his argument to your own research question and whether the students to whom Smith is referring are similar to those you are interested in.

Do I need to critically appraise all the papers I refer to in my literature review?

Although you are strongly encouraged to critically appraise the information you use throughout your literature review, less detailed critical appraisal is required in the introductory section of your literature in which you are rehearsing well-established arguments and setting the context for your own review. In this case, you do not need to do a thorough evaluation of all the evidence. You can simply cite an appropriate reference. Remember that relevant references do not have to be recent, as the example below illustrates.

In the following example, please note the reference used is for research that was undertaken several decades ago. Yet as this was seminal research for the topic in question, it is appropriate to refer back to this work.

Use of literature in your background introduction

Suppose you are doing a literature review to evaluate the perception of smokers on the health risks associated with smoking. In your introduction, you are likely to discuss what is known about the link between smoking and ill health. As this is background information to your research question, you do not need to evaluate this evidence, but can accept it at face value. You could state, for example, that 'It is well established that smoking causes lung cancer (Doll and Hill 1954)'. This is background information that is well established in the literature and you are not questioning this. It is important to note the date of this reference. As this was a seminal work, you should cite this rather than a more recent piece of work. You only need to start your critical appraisal when you begin to examine the literature that relates specifically to addressing your research question and is included in the main body of your review. However, you do need to ensure that the reference you cite is appropriate to the point you are making. If you are referring to a commonly held fact, try to trace back to the origin of this information and cite an appropriate reference, as illustrated above.

Once you have become familiar with your literature, the next step is to decide *how* you will critically appraise the literature that you have.

Critical appraisal tools

To facilitate the process of critical appraisal, there are many **critical appraisal** *tools* available to guide the evaluation of research. Critical appraisal tools are frequently used to review research, and there are many different tools available both on the Internet and in textbooks. Most of the critical appraisal tools that you encounter are designed to appraise empirical research but there are recognized approaches for evaluating the strengths and limitations of non-research papers too, although these are less well developed. You are advised to use a critical appraisal tool to assist you in the critique of your research, as it will guide you through questions you need to ask of each paper you have. It is a good practice to undertake a critical appraisal, using a recognized tool, of all of the literature you have identified for your review. Once you have identified the type of literature you have, you can select your appraisal tool.

One example of a generic (suitable for all types of academic literature) critical appraisal tool has been developed by Woolliams *et al.* (2009) and re-developed by Aveyard *et al.* (2011) (Table 5.1). These six questions to trigger critical thinking are designed to focus your thinking on the value of the literature.

The advantage of this short appraisal tool is that it can be used for any type of evidence and triggers the user to ask some elementary questions of the literature they have. It is therefore intended for use by those new to critical appraisal.

Which appraisal tool should I use?

There is a wide range of more specialized appraisal tools available. This raises the issue of which tool to use for a particular paper. Many critical appraisal tools have been specifically developed for the review of research. Some of these are generic, and suitable for all types of research – for example, Polit and Beck (2010). At first glance, you might be tempted to use a critical appraisal tool that is generic to all types of literature, especially if the literature searching strategy has identified many different types of literature that are relevant to you. However, if you can find an appraisal tool that is specific to the type of literature you have identified, this is preferable. This is because the questions will be closely related to the specific study design in question, providing an appropriate structure for the review. The questions in the design-specific appraisal tools will prompt you to ask the most relevant questions of the paper.

Table 5.1 Six questions to trigger critical thinking (adapted from Woolliams et al. 2009)

Six questions to trigger critical thinking	
Where did you find the information? • Did you just 'come across' it? Or did you access it through a systematic search?	**What** is it and **what** are the key messages or results/findings? • Is it a research study, professional opinion, discussion, website or other? • What are the key messages/results/findings?
How has the author/speaker come to their conclusions? • Is their line of reasoning logical and understandable? • If it is research or a review of research, how was it carried out, was it done well, and do the conclusions reflect the findings?	**Who** has written/said this? • Is the author/speaker an organization or individual? Are they an expert in the topic? Could they have any bias? How do you know?
When was this written/said? • Older key information may still be valid, but you need to check if there has been more recent work.	**Why** has this been written/said? • Who is the information aimed at – professionals or patient/client groups? • What is the aim of the information?

There are other critical appraisal tools that are specific to a particular research design. One set of tools has been produced by the Critical Appraisal Skills Programme (CASP), and continues to be developed by CASP International at the University of Oxford. The advantage of the CASP critical appraisal tool is that there is a specific tool for most, if not all, of the studies you are likely to encounter. CASP have published critical appraisal tools for review articles, qualitative studies, RCTs, cohort and case control studies. They are widely available on the Internet. As the websites are liable to change, a quick Google search will direct you to the latest versions of the CASP tools.

Do I have to use a critical appraisal tool?

Most researchers recommend the use of a critical appraisal tool in order to develop a consistent approach to the critique of research and other

information. Use of an appraisal tool will help you to question the literature in a more structured and in-depth way than you are likely to do
without such a tool (Florence *et al.* 2005). However, critical appraisal
tools are not without their own limitations. Take, for example, the
following research undertaken by Katrak *et al.* (2004).

Being critical of critical appraisal tools

One study identified 121 published critical appraisal tools located on the
Internet and in electronic databases (Katrak *et al.* 2004). The study found that
few of the appraisal tools had been evaluated for their effectiveness in
reviewing research or other literature. It is therefore difficult for those who
use an appraisal tool to be confident that it is 'fit for purpose'. Katrak *et al.*
concluded that there is no 'gold standard' for critical appraisal tools and that
there is a lack of information available on the development and validity of
such tools. It is important to be aware of the potential limitations of using
critical appraisal tools; however, as a novice researcher you are advised that
using an appraisal tool, which prompts you to ask questions of the literature,
is probably better than not using one.

Crowe and Sheppard (2011), following up the research of Katrak *et al.*,
came to a similar conclusion about the variable quality and validity of
published appraisal tools. In addition, Dixon-Woods *et al.* (2007) carried
out a study to compare the way in which experienced researchers
appraised a number of papers using three appraisal methods, including
use of a critical appraisal tool. They concluded that use of a critical
appraisal tool did not always lead to more consistent judgements about
the papers.

Given the limitations in the appraisal tools themselves, it could be
argued that the use of an appropriate appraisal tool to critique the
research papers is not essential, especially if you have in-depth knowledge of a particular research approach used in the paper; however, the
review process is complex and the use of an appraisal tool will assist in
the development of a systematic approach to this process and ensure
that all papers are reviewed with equal rigour. If you are reviewing the
literature for the first time and do not have an in-depth understanding of
the research approaches adopted in the studies, the use of a critical
appraisal tool is strongly recommended.

One reason for recommending the use of critical appraisal tools is that they provide a structure for you to demonstrate the rigour with which you have appraised the studies. If this adheres to your university regulations, it is recommended that you include a worked critical appraisal of each of the studies you include in your review, in the appendix of your final dissertation.

Re-emphasizing the importance of getting to know your literature

It is important to note that using a critical appraisal tool will not help you if you do not understand the fundamental principles of the research design of the study you are critiquing. It is therefore important to become familiar with the basic research methods of the research papers you have identified. If you do not understand the research methods used by the authors of the studies incorporated in your literature review, you will not be able to critique the studies with any confidence. It is therefore advisable that once you are aware of the predominant research methods that have been used by researchers studying your particular area, you develop your understanding of these methods before you begin to critique the studies. For example, if you have identified many RCTs, you are strongly advised to read about the method of undertaking RCTs before you commence your critical appraisal. Clearly, this is harder if your literature search leads you to a wide cross-section of research methods. You are not expected to develop an in-depth understanding of every research approach in the way that you would do if you had identified papers using just one or two approaches. You are advised to discuss this when writing the limitations of your study in the methods section of your literature review.

Undertaking critical appraisal of your papers for your review

The next step in the literature review process is to obtain an electronic or paper copy of the critical appraisal tools that are relevant for your research question and to begin to critically appraise each of the papers you have identified. You might find it helpful to undertake a critical appraisal of each paper and include these in an appendix of your literature review. Undertaking this process for each of your papers will serve several purposes:

- you will enhance your understanding of each paper
- you will reconsider the relevance of the paper to your review
- you will consider the strengths and weaknesses of the paper.

When you have done this, collate all the appraisals and put these together in your appendix in your final presentation of your literature review. As your understanding of the papers develops, you might find that the papers are more specific or actually discuss a different aspect of your research question than you at first thought. Be prepared to keep altering your perception of each paper. There are similarities here with the process of qualitative data analysis in which it is critical to achieve a thorough comprehension of the data before they are analysed further (Morse 1994). It is important when undertaking a literature review that you achieve this familiarity with the research and other published material that relates to your research question before you begin to combine the results of these papers.

In the following section, examples of the different approaches to the critical appraisal of the types of literature you might come across are discussed. Examples of specific appraisal tools are also given.

Critical appraisal of research

The approaches to critical appraisal of the following types of research literature will be considered:

- systematic reviews or good quality literature reviews
- quantitative studies
- qualitative studies.

How do I critique systematic reviews or good quality literature reviews?

As mentioned in Chapter 3, be wary of using systematic reviews in your literature review if they have reviewed or answered the same question as you have identified. This might mean that the work you are planning to do has already been done, unless the review was undertaken some years previously or approaches the topic from a different angle. If you come across a recent systematic review that addresses your own literature review question, you are advised to alter your question.

The first step in the critical appraisal of a review article is to determine whether or not the review has been undertaken systematically. The amount of detail given to the search, critiquing and bringing together of the evidence will differ with each literature review that has attempted to incorporate a systematic approach. The review may be described as a Cochrane or Campbell Collaboration review, in which case you can be fairly confident that it is a review that has been undertaken systematically. However, the main way to determine rigour in a review is to scrutinize the methods used to conduct the review. In all systematic reviews and good quality literature reviews, you would expect to see:

- a review question
- a methods section
- a results section
- a discussion and conclusion.

If you can identify these sections in a review (as well as a summary of them in the abstract), you can then determine whether the reviewers undertook a Cochrane or Campbell-style systematic review or a less detailed, but nonetheless systematic approach to the review. For example, a Cochrane or Campbell-style systematic review aims to uncover all literature on the topic in question, whereas a less detailed review acknowledges that the search will not be comprehensive but will identify which databases were searched. Furthermore, while a Cochrane or Campbell-style systematic review will have a team of researchers who work together in the critical analysis of the literature, a less detailed review is likely to be carried out by a single researcher with fewer resources for collaboration in these aspects. Those undertaking a systematic approach to reviewing the literature should ensure that they are explicit about the methods used to achieve this review and to demonstrate that they did everything in their power to ensure their approach was as systematic as possible.

Try not to mistake an 'information-giving' article – that may refer to lots of research findings but has not been undertaken in a systematic approach – for a systematic review or a good quality literature review. These information-giving papers may provide useful information but unless you can see how the authors searched and appraised the information they include, they do not amount to a systematic review and should not be treated as research.

Throughout this book, the rationale and process of undertaking a literature review in a systematic manner has been discussed. You will therefore be familiar with this research method and this will assist you in determining the strengths and limitations of the reviews you encounter. Authors of a review that has been approached systematically would be expected to incorporate discussion of the search strategy, method of critical appraisal and comparison of the literature, as outlined in this book.

Critical appraisal tools for systematic reviews or good quality reviews

There are several critical appraisal tools for review articles. The CASP tool for reviewing systematic reviews can be found through the CASP website. In addition, have a look at the PRISMA tool (Moher *et al.* 2009). The PRISMA tool was developed in response to concern about the poor reporting of systematic reviews in journals and is aimed at authors of reviews; however, it can be used by those who are assessing the quality of published reviews. The PRISMA tool can also be found online via a GOOGLE search.

Dealing with existing literature reviews in your review once you have commenced your study

Students undertaking a literature review are often unsure how they should proceed if they identify a systematic review in the same topic area as their own literature review once their own review is already underway. Critical appraisal is clearly vital here. One scenario is that you encounter a recently published systematic review with the same focus as your own literature review. Ask yourself the following two questions of the review.

Has the review been undertaken systematically?

Assess the quality of the review, to determine whether it is a systematic review or more of a narrative review. If there is no explicitly recorded method of how the literature was searched, critiqued and analysed, then the review is less likely to be of high quality and it may be appropriate to proceed with a systematic approach to the question in your own literature review.

How recent is the review?

If critical appraisal of the systematic review identifies a very recent, good quality review and this is encountered early on in your course of study, it would be wise to alter the question slightly so as to avoid direct repetition of the review question. You could be penalized for lack of originality and it could be difficult to demonstrate that the review was undertaken in a thorough and independent way without relying on ideas that were found already published in another review. However, if the systematic review is identified once you are already immersed in the literature review process and a change of question is not desirable, this should be fully documented in the methods section of your literature review. You should then make an extra effort to ensure that the originality of your work is established and that the methods of searching, critiquing and analysing the literature are clearly documented so that it is clear that the results you present are your own work. You may however use the reference list of the systematic review to ensure that the literature included in your own literature review is comprehensive.

If a systematic review is encountered that is a direct repetition of your review question, but was published a few years previously, you can use this as the background to your own review and focus on providing an update to the review that already exists. Whitlock *et al.* (2008) suggest that reviews are often out of date within three to five years or even less. If you consider the existing review to be of high quality, your search strategy can reflect this, commencing at the point at which the original systematic review ceased to search for literature. With a reduced time span over which to search, you will have more time to search wider and deeper for materials that are harder to access. This will improve the quality of your work. If the review is recent and of good quality, you may consider your question has been answered.

How do I critique quantitative studies?

Most quantitative studies that you will encounter fall into one of the following categories: RCT (or similar trial), case control study, cohort study or **cross-sectional study** using questionnaire/surveys. One of the main approaches to assessing the quality of quantitative work is to assess the validity and reliability of the study. Validity refers to whether the study measures what it intends to measure, and reliability refers to whether the measurement is reliable and would yield the same results on repeated measurements. There are CASP critical appraisal tools for RCTs, cohort studies and case control trials.

Your critical appraisal of quantitative studies will be greatly assisted if you are familiar with the particular research method used in the study. This can be difficult for those who encounter a wide range of literature, as a novice researcher cannot be expected to have in-depth knowledge of all research methods. However, those who find that their search strategy leads them to papers incorporating one or two research methods are advised to develop their understanding of these particular methods. To assist your understanding of each study that you have identified, the following questions can be asked of each quantitative paper.

What is the journal of publication?

Those reviewing quantitative research should be aware of the quality of the journal in which the research is published. In principle, a journal is considered to be of good quality if it is peer-reviewed; that is, each paper is reviewed by at least one recognized expert in the subject area about which the paper is written, prior to acceptance for publication in the journal. However, it should be noted that the peer-review process is not perfect. Papers are generally considered by one or two experts in a field and it is not possible for an expert to know every aspect about any particular topic. Occasionally, corrections or amendments to a paper appear in later publications of the journal. In reality, the peer-review process takes place when the research paper is published!

What is the research question and why was the study conducted?

The study question should be clear and should be founded on argument and rationale as to why the study was undertaken. The study should be appropriate for quantitative study; that is, the results should be measurably numerical.

What method was selected to undertake the research?

In most papers there will be a short summary of the research process undertaken and from this you will be able to identify how the study was conducted. See if you can identify the type of study and compare the methods used with those described in the research methods textbooks.

How big was the sample?

The sample refers to those who took part in the study. The sample is taken from a wider population to whom the research project relates. For example, a sample of university students could be taken from the university population as a whole. Sample size in quantitative research tends to be large. This is because researchers are concerned with validity; that is, whether the findings of a study are valid or reflect reality. For example, you are likely to have greater confidence in a study comparing two treatment options in which many thousands of people had participated than a study conducted on just 20 participants. However, if the condition under investigation is unusual, sample sizes inevitably will be smaller. The authors of quantitative research papers should demonstrate how they determined the sample size for the research in question. This should be clearly documented in the paper and is often referred to as a 'power calculation'.

Has the appropriate sample been obtained?

You need to question who was selected to participate in the study. Be careful to identify if the study was carried out on a certain group of people, as this may not be representative of the wider population. For example, a study might suggest that it is exploring nurses' attitudes to euthanasia but when you look closely at the sample, only a small group of nurses working in palliative care were consulted.

How were the data collected?

The data collection method should be appropriate for the study design. Quantitative research often uses a wide variety of data collection methods for attributes that are appropriate for objective measurement. If the data were collected using a questionnaire and there is a low response rate, you can question the validity of the findings.

How were the data analysed?

Quantitative data are usually analysed statistically, as described in Chapter 3, and you should expect to find reference to the statistical tests used in the paper in order to make sense of the data.

Critical appraisal tools for quantitative studies

Randomized controlled trials

In addition to the specific CASP appraisal tools, there are further resources for those reviewing quantitative studies. Those reviewing RCTs are advised to refer to the **CONSORT statement**. The CONSORT (Consolidated Standards of Reporting Trials) statement was issued in 1996 and revised in 2001, 2008 and 2010 (Schulz *et al.* 2010). The CONSORT statement was issued in response to concern about the quality of the reporting of RCTs submitted for publication. There was concern that without thorough and transparent reporting of the process of conducting RCTs, the quality of the trials could not be assessed. The CONSORT statement comprises a checklist and flow diagram to enable both the researchers and those reviewing the research to identify good practice in the conduct and presentation of RCTs. The aim of the CONSORT statement is to make the process of undertaking and publishing RCTs as clear as possible, so that users of the research can evaluate the strengths and limitations of the study. The CONSORT statement gives clear guidance to researchers concerning which aspects of the design of the RCT they should make explicit to readers of the research, to ensure that those who read and use the research have clear information concerning the way in which the RCT was conducted. Schulz *et al.* (2010) provide full details of the revised CONSORT statement. The statement includes discussion of the scientific background for the study, eligibility of participants and interventions intended for each group, random allocation and blinding, statistical analysis and discussion of results.

Cohort and case control studies

For those reviewing *cohort studies*, Rochon *et al.* (2005) have identified factors relevant to the quality of such studies. These can be used in conjunction with the CASP critical appraisal tool for cohort studies. Rochon *et al.* recommend that the following aspects of the trial are taken into consideration. First, assess how the comparison was made between the groups. This includes how the groups were selected and how they were defined. Second, consider whether the comparison makes sense; in other words, whether a cohort study was a useful method of studying the research topic. Third, consider any potential selection biases. The important difference between an RCT and a cohort study is that in an RCT there are two or more groups that are allocated at random. Each group receives a different treatment and the differences in outcome can be attributed to the treatment given, as the groups were allocated at random and therefore considered equal in all other respects. In a cohort study, the cohort and control group are not allocated at random but arise naturally in the population. For example, those who use illicit drugs might be a naturally occurring cohort group. This group of illicit drug users can then be compared with non-users at the end of the trial. Any differences between the two groups cannot be attributed to the exposure or intervention given, as the cohort and control groups were never equal.

For those reviewing *case control studies*, Crombie (2006) suggests that the following essential questions are asked of them. How were the cases obtained? Was the control group appropriate? Were the data collected in the same way for cases as for controls?

Questionnaires and surveys

For those reviewing *cross-sectional studies – surveys/questionnaires*, there is a classic text (Oppenheim, 1992) entitled *Questionnaire Design, Interviewing and Attitude Measurement*. If you have many questionnaire survey studies to appraise, you are well advised to become familiar with these principles of questionnaire design.

Greenhalgh (2010) comments on the ease with which a poor quality questionnaire can be produced without due regard to the process of ensuring that the questionnaire will facilitate the collection of useful data. She discusses the frequent use of poorly designed questionnaires that lack rigour and hence lead to the collection of poor quality data and subsequently to misleading conclusions.

Greenhalgh suggests ten questions to ask about papers that describe questionnaire research:

Ten questions to ask about papers that describe the results of questionnaires

Was the question appropriate to a questionnaire design?

Was the questionnaire tool valid and reliable?

What did the questionnaire look like?

Were the instructions clear?

Was it piloted?

Who was the sample?

How was it administered?

How were the data analysed?

What were the results?

What were the conclusions?

(Greenhalgh 2010)

These questions are explained as follows: once you have established if the research question was suitable for questionnaire research (many sensitive topics may be better suited to in-depth interviews), the main issue to consider is whether the questionnaire has been tested for validity and reliability. A questionnaire will only collect useful data if the questions have been well tested and piloted. This is to ensure that the questions mean the same thing to those who respond as they do to those who designed them. This will also include how the questions are presented. Even with the best designed questionnaire, unless it is distributed to a representative sample of the population, the quality of the results will be reduced. A postal questionnaire can be distributed to a random sample of the population; however, it is highly unlikely that everyone will respond. This affects the quality of the data, as it is not known how the responses from those who did not respond would have differed from those who did.

Alternatively, if it is possible to distribute a questionnaire face to face, you may achieve a higher response rate, but you will not achieve a random sample, as you are only selecting participants from those patients/clients attending on a particular day. For example, if you distributed the questionnaire in a shopping centre on a Saturday, you would reach a different population than if the questionnaire was distributed on a weekday. Similarly, you would be likely to get a different group of people depending on the time at which the questionnaire was distributed. Thus, it is very difficult to achieve a random sample in a questionnaire survey that is distributed face to face, as only those in attendance on that day have the possibility of responding to the questionnaire. It is equally very difficult to achieve a random sample in a postal questionnaire as the response rates tend to be low. For these reasons and due to the difficulty of creating a questionnaire that measures what you intend to measure, the quality of data obtained from questionnaires will be affected by the methods used and needs to be carefully considered in each case.

In summary, for those critiquing quantitative research, there are two main objectives. First, you should become as familiar as possible with the research approach undertaken in the study. Second, you should apply this knowledge when reviewing the rigour of the study by using an appropriate critical appraisal tool.

How do I critique qualitative studies?

Are qualitative studies appraised differently from quantitative studies?

There has been much discussion in recent years concerning the ways in which qualitative research is evaluated and this debate is ongoing. With the advent of evidence-based practice and the need to demonstrate accountability in research, there has been increasing demand for evidence of rigour in qualitative research. Clearly, without evidence of rigour in the undertaking of the study, the worth of any study can be questioned. However, the search for evidence of rigour in qualitative research is difficult due to the interpretative and exploratory nature of qualitative studies. It can therefore be difficult for those who critique a qualitative study to determine the strengths and limitations of the study. This is because qualitative studies typically do not seek to quantify or measure the items under exploration using numbers – an approach that lies traditionally in the quantitative domain, in which the measurements taken by the researchers are repeatable and re-testable. In contrast, most qualitative studies use exploratory interviews, focus groups or observations in order to collect a rich data set, which can then be analysed qualitatively; that is, by exploring emerging themes rather than by statistics.

The aim of most qualitative data analysis is to study the interview scripts or other data obtained for the study and to develop an understanding of these data. The data are coded and themes are then generated from the data set. The generation of themes, although rigorous, is interpretative and subjective, depending on the insight of the researcher. Qualitative data analysis is therefore open to interpretation. Because the researcher is involved in, and indeed shapes, both the data collection and analysis process, it is not possible for the researcher to remain detatched from the data collected. It is also not desirable to strive for such a detatchment. The richness of qualitative enquiry arises from the dialogue between the researcher and the researched, and the insights obtained through this process are only possible because of the interaction between the two.

The interviewer may probe the interviewee about his or her responses to a question and so phrases the next question as a direct response to the reply received. The richness of the data is dependent on the interaction between the researcher and researched and the process is necessarily subjective. Subjectivity is required for the researcher to get an insight into the topic of investigation and objectivity is not strived for.

The concept of reflexivity refers to the acknowledgement by the qualitative researcher that the process of enquiry is necessarily open to interpretation and that detachment from the focus of the research is neither desirable nor possible. Guba and Lincoln (1995) reinforce this argument by describing the construction of the findings of qualitative research – constructed by the dialogue between the researcher and the researched.

What does a good qualitative study look like?

For the reasons outlined, there has been much debate about how the strengths and limitations of a qualitative study can be determined. Concern has long been expressed about qualitative research being subject to the same criteria for reliability and validity as quantitative studies (Lincoln and Guba 1985; Horsburgh 2003). Horsburgh (2003) argues that if qualitative research is judged by the same standard as quantitative research, then the impression may be created that qualitative research is not academically rigorous. Yet, qualitative researchers adhere to procedures that ensure rigour throughout the research process.

As discussed in an earlier section, the quality of quantitative work is often assessed for the validity and reliability of the study. Because the 'measurements' obtained in qualitative research are made through the interpretation of the researchers, most qualitative researchers argue that it is not possible to assess qualitative research in the same way as quantitative research. For this reason, Lincoln and Guba (1985) argue that the terms 'credibility', '**transferability**', 'dependability' and 'confirmability' are more appropriate for assessing the quality of a qualitative study than terms such as 'validity' and 'reliability'. They argue that all qualitative research should have a 'truth value' and that this could be determined by strategies that represent the hallmark of good qualitative research, such as keeping an accurate trail of the research process and transparency in the data analysis process.

Yet, despite concern about the appropriate way to assess the quality of qualitative research, not all researchers agree with Lincoln and Guba's (1985) approach to the assessment of quality in qualitative research. Morse *et al.* (2002) argue that the approach advocated by Lincoln and Guba is unhelpful, as it encourages researchers to review the quality of the research at the end of the research process rather than to keep re-evaluating the quality of the research process as the research is ongoing. Morse argues that the terms 'validity' and 'reliability' are appropriate to qualitative research and cites Kvale (1989), who argues that validity means to investigate, to check and to question – all of which are necessary components of any quality assessment of qualitative research. Indeed, you will often find the term validity applied to qualitative research (Greenhalgh 2010), indicating that there is no consensus about the terms used.

It is important for those who review qualitative research to be aware that there is also no consensus among qualitative researchers about what constitutes a good qualitative study, how a study is critiqued or the terminology to be used when referring to both qualitative studies and critiquing tools (Popay *et al.* 1998; Sandelowski and Barroso 2002; Russell and Gregory 2003; Shin *et al.* 2009). Consequently, you are likely to encounter a variety of qualitative research incorporating a wide range of approaches and methods, and an equally wide variety of appraisal tools for the critique of qualitative research. You need to be aware of these tensions so that you are not confused by the different approaches and rationale when these are encountered. It is also important that you are familiar with the basic principles of qualitative research and how the approach differs from quantitative research, so that you can assess the individual quality of the research you encounter.

Critical appraisal of qualitative studies

Not withstanding the above, the following principles can be used to critique qualitative studies.

Who wrote the paper?

In qualitative research, it is particularly important that the researchers have the necessary experience to undertake the research. This is because in qualitative research the quality of the data collected is dependent on the skills of the researcher. Qualitative research is reflexive, which means that the researcher's own values, experience and interests shape the research process. The researcher interacts with the participants in order to get as much insight into the research topic as possible and, therefore, the best quality data. The researcher may ask probing questions to get richer data on a particular aspect of the topic and the way that this is done reflects the experience and expertise of the researcher. Therefore, questions that can be asked of the author include their relevant qualifications and experience and whether they have the necessary insight into the topic area to address the research question.

Where is the paper published?

Those reviewing qualitative research need to be aware of the accredited quality of the journal in which the research is published. As mentioned previously, you should consider whether the journal is peer-reviewed.

Is there a research question and is the method appropriate for addressing the question?

Qualitative research will commence with an identified research question and the method chosen to address the question should be appropriate to this. For example, if the research question is exploratory – *'How do people who are homeless describe their experience living in a hostel?'* – then the method of answering the question should also be explorative, as is appropriate for qualitative study. In Chapter 2, a brief introduction to the different approaches to qualitative research was outlined. Those reviewing qualitative research should be familiar with the different approaches so that they can identify why a particular approach has been adopted in any research study. For example, researchers who are interested in exploring participants' experience of being homeless might adopt a phenomenological approach to their research. However, a phenomenological approach would not be appropriate for someone interested in exploring the attitudes of those who are homeless, as this type of study is concerned with exploring the lived experience only, rather than attitudes related to this. An appropriate approach to exploring the lived experience of people who are homeless might be to interview people who have had this experience. It would not be appropriate to observe people who are homeless, as this would not achieve an insight into the way in which they would describe their experience. Thus, it is important that the method chosen to address the question is appropriate to the research question itself.

Was the right qualitative research method used?

The data collection method selected should also be appropriate to the method and research question. The most commonly used data collection methods in qualitative research are in-depth interviews, focus groups and observation. Those reviewing qualitative research reports should assess how the data collection methods were determined and the appropriateness of these to the research question. In-depth interviews are used when the insight into a particular topic is sought from the participant. The interviewer will be trained and skilled in asking questions that probe the experience of the participant and the aim is to generate rich data through one-to-one dialogue. Focus groups are a form of group interview and may be selected over in-depth interviews when dialogue between research participants – rather than in-depth discussion with one participant – is regarded as a positive contribution to the study. For example, if the research topic is unfamiliar to those involved and participants may not have developed their thoughts in relation to this topic, focus groups can be useful as a data collection method as the ideas expressed by one participant may trigger a response in another participant. However, if a topic is particularly sensitive, participants may be reluctant to express their thoughts in a focus group and in-depth interviews may be more appropriate.

The role of questionnaires in the collection of qualitative data should be mentioned at this point. While it is possible to collect qualitative data through open-ended questions on a questionnaire schedule, such data are not likely to be as in-depth as that collected through one-to-one interaction. Therefore, when a qualitative research study incorporates a questionnaire survey into its methods, the quality of the qualitative data collected should be considered carefully. Data collected through observation are especially useful when actual observations are sought rather than participants' interpretations. For example, the extent to which nurses comply with infection control policies can be measured more accurately through direct observation than any other method, as it is well known that participants may not accurately self-report their behaviour. It is important to note that observational data may be used in both quantitative and qualitative studies. For example, the number of infection control practices undertaken by each practitioner could be counted numerically, or the nature of the interaction between practitioner and patient could be observed using qualitative approaches. Therefore, when reviewing a qualitative study, you should make an assessment as to the appropriateness of the method used in the study in addressing the research question.

What was the sample for the study?

Most qualitative researchers use purposive sampling rather than random sampling in their research. It is important to be aware of the differences between the two. A random sample is where participants are picked at random from the population being studied and every person in that population has an equal chance of being selected. For example, a random sample of students could be identified if a computer identified students at random from a register. In purposive sampling, an appropriate sample from the population is chosen according to particular criteria. Participants are chosen for their suitability to provide rich data for in-depth study. For this reason, random sampling would be inappropriate, as it may fail to identify information-rich participants. Thus, any qualitative study that uses random sampling rather than purposive sampling should cause you to question why this particular approach was adopted. You should also consider the type of participant who makes up the purposive sample. For example, if the researchers are exploring people who are homeless, then a purposive sample obtained in Glasgow is likely to be very different to a sample from London. Similarly, the characteristics of a sample are likely to vary depending on the particular area in Glasgow from which the sample is drawn. This will affect the extent to which the results are transferable from one context to another and, therefore, the relevance of the particular research study to the literature review question.

An alternative sampling strategy that might be used in qualitative research is theoretical sampling. Theoretical sampling is an approach commonly used in grounded theory in which the sample is identified as the study progresses, according to the needs of the study. Another sampling strategy is snowball sampling, in which the sample is developed as new potential participants are identified as the study progresses. For example, the contacts of participants already involved in the research may be invited to enter the study, if they have the relevant experience. You would expect to find purposive, theoretical or snowball sampling used in a qualitative study.

How big was the sample?

Sample sizes in qualitative research tend to be small. The sample should be large enough to achieve sufficient information-rich cases for in-depth data analysis, but not so large that the amount of data obtained becomes unmanageable. A small sample is required because in-depth understanding (rather than statistical analysis) is sought from information-rich participants who take part. For this reason, a small sample size should be regarded as appropriate in qualitative research. This is in contrast to quantitative research in which the nearer the sample size is to the true population, the more representative the results will be. Russell and Gregory (2003) argue that different qualitative approaches require different sample sizes and advise that phenomenological studies tend to have smaller samples than grounded theory studies or ethnographic studies. When you are reviewing a study, it is important to consider the account given by the researchers of the way in which the sample size was arrived at throughout the course of any study.

How were the data collected?

The way in which the data were collected should also be considered. Most researchers advocate that in-depth interviews and focus groups should be recorded so that the interviews can be transcribed word for word. However, some researchers argue that this is time-consuming and that the time could be better used by undertaking additional interviews and hence collecting considerably more data. There are many variations in the way that qualitative data may be collected. For example, some researchers advocate that interview transcripts are returned to the participants in order that the participants check and validate the content of the transcript for accuracy. However, other researchers argue that this is time-consuming and unnecessarily burdensome on participants who may not remember the interview or who may not wish to revisit the content of the interview they gave (Barbour 2001). They may also wish to alter the content of the interview, thus affecting its validity. It is important that the researchers justify the approach they have taken to the data collection process and can demonstrate that the process was undertaken systematically and rigorously.

How were the data analysed?

The reviewer should consider the way in which the method of data analysis is reported in a qualitative research study. Although word restrictions impose limitations on the detail that can be given in any journal paper, there should be evidence of a considered approach to data analysis. Use of a computer package may be evident, but this in itself does not ensure rigour in the analysis process. Equally, it is possible to demonstrate rigour in data analysis without the use of computer packages. There might also be justification as to how much data had been collected and whether saturation was achieved. Data saturation means that at the end of the analysis period, the continuing data analysis does not identify additional new themes, but instead the data that are analysed merely add to the existing themes that have emerged from previous data analysis.

In summary, critical appraisal of qualitative research papers is complex and while novice researchers are expected to be aware of the complexities and many different approaches to undertaking qualitative studies, they are not expected to offer a contribution to the debate. Those reviewing qualitative research should become familiar with the particular approaches to qualitative study that have been used in the papers they have identified. They should then assess the rigour of the papers with the aid of a critical appraisal tool.

Critical appraisal tools for qualitative studies

The diverse nature of qualitative research means that it is often difficult to critique, especially for a novice researcher. It is also argued that it is difficult to find an appraisal tool that is appropriate for every qualitative research paper encountered. Barbour (2001) argues that the vast diversity of qualitative methods means that the critique of any qualitative paper by means of a simple checklist or appraisal tool can be difficult. However, the benefits of using a critical appraisal tool rather than using an unstructured approach have also been highlighted. You are therefore advised to use a tool when appraising qualitative research but to be aware of the limitations of doing so and also to be aware that the tool may not be appropriate for every such piece of research.

There are a variety of critical appraisal tools available and an Internet search will enable you to view many of those accessible. As outlined above, because of the complexity of the topic, there is no one tool that is best for all qualitative research; however, one commonly used appraisal tool is the CASP qualitative critical appraisal tool, available on the CASP website. Other useful resources for students include the guide to critiquing qualitative studies found in the research methods textbook of Polit and Beck (2010) as well as Greenhalgh (2010). There are also the Consolidated Criteria for Reporting Qualitative Research (COREQ) (Tong *et al.* 2007).

In summary, you are advised to use a critical appraisal tool – rather than no tool at all – and whichever tool is selected, it is very important that you are familiar with the general principles of qualitative research, as outlined in Chapter 3, so that you can apply the appraisal tool appropriately to any given study. Some general principles to assist with the critical appraisal are given below.

How do I critique theory?

Earlier in this book it was suggested that you are unlikely to need to appraise theory, as it is unlikely to be a main component of your review. However, if your research question does require you to evaluate theory, here are some points to bear in mind. The term 'theory' means different things to different people. We use the term in different ways. Sometimes we use it loosely and might say '*I have a theory about why that man was murdered*'. In this case, your theory is speculation. Other theories are far more developed and refer to a detailed explanation about the way things happen or are expected to happen. Take, for example, Darwin's theory of evolution, which he wrote after studying the way in which animals and humans seem to have evolved. You will be aware that this theory is often challenged, and without concrete evidence it remains just a theory. We do not know for certain that this is the way man evolved. Often in health and social care, a theory is developed as a result of research findings. Another example is Prochaska and colleagues' (1994) stages of change model mentioned in Chapters 2 and 3. The authors looked at the evidence behind the way in which people change behaviour and wrote their theory, which seemed a reasonable way to incorporate what we know about the ways in which people change behaviour. However, again, this remains just a theory and others have challenged this explanation (see, for example, West 2006), arguing that there is evidence that some people make snap decisions about behaviour change without following all the stages outlined in the stages of change model.

It is therefore important that when you come across a theory, you do not accept it at face value. It might be little more than someone's speculation, and so you need to appraise the theory. Woolliams and colleagues' (2009) appraisal tool cited above would be a useful tool with which to begin the appraisal in order to ask questions of the theory development. In particular, the following questions are central: who wrote the theory and what is the evidence behind the ideas promoted in the theory?

How do I critique practice literature?

Practice literature can be any literature based in the practice area that falls short of research. Those using practice-based evidence in their literature review need to identify how they are going to assess the quality of this information, in the same way as they would consider the quality of primary research or a systematic review, although tools developed for research (for example, the CASP tools) would not normally be used for non-research literature. You will find any generic critical appraisal tool, such as Cottrell (2005) and Woolliams et al. (2009) useful. You need to make judgements about the quality of practice literature in order to assess how much weight it should carry in your review. For example, a discussion article written by a leading expert in a particular area might be considered to carry more weight than a similar article written by a student.

Hek et al. (2000) report the following criteria for critiquing non-research articles:

- Is the subject relevant to the review question?
- Is it accurate?
- Is it well written and credible?
- Is it peer-reviewed in any way?
- Does it ring true?
- In what quality of journal is the report published?

Reviewers are also encouraged to examine the following attributes of a paper to determine the quality of the information provided: the intended target audience, credentials of the author, the publisher of the information and the way in which the information is presented; that is, the extent to which the author is suitably qualified to report on the topic in question should be examined. Similarly, an article would carry more weight if it were published in an academic journal rather than in a newspaper.

However, it is important to remember that the expert opinion of a well-known figure in the area might be found to contradict established findings from empirical research. For example, in recent discussions about climate change, many experts have been consulted about their perception of current signs of climate change. However, in the absence of empirical evidence, the validity of their opinion can only be speculated. It should be noted that information obtained from websites might be critically appraised using this approach.

Critical appraisal of an argument

Another approach to reviewing the quality of a non-empirical research paper in which arguments are presented is to assess the quality of the arguments presented in the paper. This approach was originally advocated by Thouless and Thouless (1953), who discuss the use of logic in the constructed argument presented in a discussion paper. They articulate 38 'dishonest tricks' commonly used in argument, including:

- using emotionally charged words
- making statements using words such as 'all' when 'some' would be more appropriate
- using selected instances
- misrepresentation of opposing arguments
- evasion of a sound refutation of an argument.

You are also advised to consult the 15-item checklist devised by Cottrell (2005) for the evaluation of an academic essay. You can also use Woolliams and colleagues' (2009) critical appraisal checklist. Criteria include whether the conclusion is clear and based on evidence, whether the arguments are well structured and presented in a logical order, whether good use is made of alternative arguments and whether these are referenced.

Those reviewing discussion articles and expert opinions are encouraged to scrutinize the way in which the article is written as a guide to the strength of argument presented. Reviewers should question the use of language, the acknowledgement of alternative approaches or lines of argument, forced analogy, false credentials, and so on. Does the evidence on which the arguments are founded bear scrutiny? If the arguments are well constructed and defensible, then greater weight can be given to these arguments than those that are less well prepared and constructed.

Which one has greater credibility?
Consider George Monbiot's (2005) response to David Bellamy in *The Guardian* regarding the evidence behind the environmental threat presented by global warming. George Monbiot refers to recent research findings to reinforce his argument while David Bellamy argues from his opinion only. If you applied Thouless and Thouless's (1953) criteria to these arguments, which one would have greater credibility?

How do I appraise policy and guidelines?

As discussed earlier in this book, unless the focus of your review is evaluating the use of policy or guidelines in a particular area, you are unlikely to need to appraise guidelines in detail in the main body of your review; you are more likely to refer to them in the introduction or discussion sections of your review in reference to your main findings. Guidelines and policy documents are generally produced either locally or nationally. As with all literature that you include in your review, do not assume that they will be valid or based on reliable evidence until you have reviewed them in detail. Ideally, guidelines and policy should be based on the best available evidence and the first thing you need to do is establish the evidence base upon which the guidelines and policies are based. If this is not clear, then this is an obvious limitation of the policy or guidelines. Guidelines and policies documents can then be reviewed using the generic critical appraisal checklists (Cottrell 2005; Woolliams *et al.* 2009).

The Agree Collaboration offers guidance for the development of guidelines and also a critical appraisal tool for assessing the quality of guidelines and policy. The AGREE 11 tool is available at http://www.agreecollaboration.org/.

How do I appraise information on websites?

The Internet contains a wealth of information that may be useful for health and social care practitioners. Indeed, there is even evidence that Internet searches can be used by health and social care professionals for the benefit of their patients and clients (Giustini 2005; Tang and Ng 2006).

However, it has to be acknowledged that websites are unregulated and it is possible for anybody to publish anything on an Internet site. You are therefore recommended to be critical of any websites you encounter. Fink (2005) suggests that you should ask the following questions of any websites you encounter:

- Who supports the site?
- When was it last updated?
- What authority do the authors of the site have?

If you are happy with the answers you get to these questions, any material you encounter on a website can be subjected to the critical appraisal strategies as advocated by Hek *et al.* (2000), Thouless and Thouless (1953) and Cottrell (2005).

Information from websites is unlikely to be research papers, unless of course you are searching an academic **database** on which academic papers are available online. Information on websites will likely to relate to practice and policy literature. While it is possible and necessary to critique the quality of this information incorporated into a review, it is important to remember that non-research articles do not usually represent strong evidence upon which to draw conclusions. Non-research articles should be appraised using the generic guidelines suggested above and incorporated into the study, while acknowledging the limitations inherent in the evidence they give.

What next, now that I have critically appraised all my literature?

At this point, you will have written detailed critical appraisals for each of the research papers or other literature you have identified for your review. As a result, you will have an in-depth knowledge of your studies and be aware of the strengths and weaknesses of each study and the extent to which it contributes to your understanding of your literature review question.

Rejecting irrelevant papers

If you have any papers that seemed relevant on the initial review of the abstract but no longer seem relevant to your research question following in-depth critical appraisal, these should be discarded at this point.

Finding the core or main papers

You may find that one or a few papers stand out as particularly relevant or important to your research question. It might be that the methods used are particularly robust or the findings are comprehensive and relate to a lot of aspects of the literature review question that you have. Or the paper might be one of a series of papers by researchers who have done a lot of work in the area. These 'core' papers are useful as they can provide an initial focus to your analysis, as we will see in the next chapter. Have a look through your papers and the critical appraisals of the papers and see if any stand out in this way.

Preparation for developing themes

Once you have critically appraised all your papers, you are ready to start the next stage of your analysis, which is developing themes – which we discuss in the next chapter.

Tips for doing your critique of the literature

1 Undertake a critical appraisal on all of the literature that you have identified for your review. This will ensure that you really get to know your literature.
2 Remember that to critique means to give the positive and negative points about a paper. You are not expected only to be negative. Emphasize the good points about the paper. But no research is perfect!
3 Remember to describe the critical appraisal tools you use. Be explicit about the way you appraised the information, including non-research papers.
4 Consider putting a copy of each critique in the appendix of your presentation of your literature review, if the regulations of your academic institution permit.

In summary

When you critique the literature you have identified for your review, you need to focus on the following questions:

1 Is this literature relevant to my review?
2 Have I identified literature at the top of my hierarchy of evidence?
3 Have I identified the strengths and weaknesses of these papers and am aware of their relevance to my review question?

It is important to be aware that the quality of information you may encounter will vary widely. You should carry out a critical appraisal of all the sources you include in your literature review and you should be able to discuss with confidence the relevance and strengths and limitations of your literature to your research question. It is good practice to complete a critical appraisal tool for each piece of evidence you include and incorporate this in the appendix of your literature review. The purpose of critical appraisal is to determine the relevance, strengths and limitations of the information collected so that you can determine the weight each paper should have in answering the research question. A study might be well-carried out but not specific enough to address your research question. Alternatively, a study might be very relevant to your research question but not well designed or implemented. Furthermore, non-empirical information might add interesting insight to your argument, but the quality of this information also needs to be assessed. Without this critical appraisal, the contribution of this evidence to addressing the research question cannot be assessed. The final stage of your literature review is to combine the evidence and present your findings. This is addressed in the next chapter.

Key points

- Critical appraisal is a necessary process in determining the relevance, appropriateness and quality of the published information related to your research question.
- The first step in the critical appraisal process is to read and re-read your papers.
- You need to distinguish between papers that report empirical findings and those that present discussion or expert opinion only.
- You are advised to use one of the many critical appraisal tools that are available to structure your critical appraisal.
- A critical appraisal tool will not help you unless you understand what your paper is about before you start to appraise.

6

How do I analyse my findings?

Developing your themes

The critical appraisal of each paper is the first stage of the analysis process in a literature review. The next stage is the development of themes from the findings or results section of each of your papers, bearing in mind the strengths and weaknesses of the papers you have already identified. In this chapter, we discuss how you begin to develop themes that address your literature review question.

Which papers should I include?

The first thing to consider is how much good quality research literature (assuming research literature is what you need) addresses your research question. Think back to your inclusion criteria, developed from your own hierarchy of evidence and identify how much evidence you have. The following guidelines refer to those undertaking an undergraduate degree and are intended as a rough guide only.

- If you have approximately ten good quality research papers that are relevant to your research, then include these ten papers and exclude any remaining research papers that you have assessed as less relevant to your research question.
- If you have only five good quality papers that are directly relevant, then include these five but consider including the papers that you have assessed as less relevant or less good quality. In your methods section of your dissertation, explain that you are aware that they are less relevant or of poorer quality but there was an insufficient number of better quality/relevant papers.
- If you have two research papers that are directly relevant/good quality and three that are indirectly relevant/less good quality, you might consider using some of the non-research literature that is relevant to your research question – for example, **discussion papers** or expert opinion. In this case, these non-research papers can be considered to be the 'next best thing' to research, given that there is a lack of research. You also need to consider how you will deal with expert opinion that goes against the main flow of your research evidence. It is important to acknowledge this opinion but state that as the evidence it provides is not strong, this literature will not weigh heavily in your review. What is

important is that you are aware of the limitations of the literature you include and you are explicit about this.

Why do some reviews reject papers on the basis of quality even if there is little evidence available?

This is an interesting point. Some systematic review protocols require researchers to make a judgement about the quality of each paper and include only literature that meets specified quality indicator criteria in their review, irrespective of the amount of research they have found. Thus it is possible for a systematic review team to find 20 papers but to reject all but three, having assessed 17 papers as of insufficient quality for inclusion in the review. The implication of this is that the review contains only high-quality evidence and omits literature of poorer quality. You can see the strengths and weaknesses of this approach. On the positive side, if only high-quality evidence is included, then you might have more confidence in the findings of the review. On the negative side, the papers not included might contribute to answering the research question in some way, as outlined above. Clearly, no review is perfect and those doing a review must make methodological decisions along the way and justify these when they write up their review.

Considerations of quality in qualitative research

Notwithstanding the above, there is discussion in the research literature about whether qualitative research should be excluded from a review on the basis of quality. Some researchers (Bondas and Hall 2007; Noyes and Popay 2007; Finlayson and Dixon 2008; Thomas and Harden 2008) included all qualitative studies within their literature review, but acknowledged the quality of the studies included. On the other hand, Walsh and Downe (2005), Caroll *et al.* (2010) and Harden (2007) all reported using indicators of quality to exclude qualitative studies from their literature review. The difficulty arises, as discussed in Chapter 5, in that there is no strong consensus regarding what constitutes quality in a qualitative study, so attempts to reject papers on the basis of quality can be difficult to make.

Combining the evidence

The next step is to summarize the findings of your literature review into manageable amounts. However, you are aiming to achieve more than just a summary of your results. The aim is to interpret the results. This will allow you to consider why one study obtained a different set of results from those obtained by a similar study, and how the results of each study were shaped by the methods used to collect the data. You are seeking to explain the differences and similarities in the different papers that you have, rather than to simply summarize them. The goal is to 'produce a new and integrative interpretation of findings that is more substantive than those resulting from individual investigation' (Finfgeld 2003, p. 894).

The aim is to bring together the different studies or other pieces of information and to find new meaning from the sum of these papers viewed as a whole rather than that which could be obtained by reading each paper individually.

This might seem a daunting task, but if it is tackled in a step-by-step manner, as this chapter illustrates, it will become manageable. Importantly, it is this process that makes your literature review original and unique. The discoveries and insights you make as you compare and contrast the literature are only possible because you have followed the systematic process of identifying and reviewing the published information relating to your topic. They are a testament to your developing skills as a researcher.

There are many different approaches to bringing this information together and there is much debate about how this should be done. One common term for this process is **meta-synthesis**. Meta-synthesis is described as the science of 'summing up' (Light and Pillemer 1984) and is described by Finlayson and Dixon (2008), Bondas and Hall (2007), Walsh and Downe (2005) and Rice (2008). Other terms to describe this process include 'meta-aggregative approach' (Hannes and Lockwood 2011), 'thematic synthesis' (Thomas and Harden 2008), 'meta-ethnography', 'meta-study' and 'meta-narrative' (Barnett-Page and Thomas 2009).

There are many find different ideas about bringing qualitative research together. Some qualitative researchers have argued that it is not appropriate to attempt to bring together the results of research studies at all; to do so is to strip the work of the depth and insight that it gives and that, as a consequence, all qualitative research should stand alone rather than be combined (Sandelowski *et al.* 1997). Yet, if qualitative research is considered to be generalizable (Morse 1999), then the results have to be viewed in relation to others. Other researchers argue that only papers that have been undertaken using a particular research methodology can be compared (Jensen and Allen 1996). The principles of meta-analysis, for example (as referred to in the section below), require that only the results of studies that have used similar methods can be combined to be re-analysed statistically. Jensen and Allen (1996) have applied this principle to qualitative research and argue that qualitative research studies using phenomenology could be combined but that the results of a phenomenological study and a grounded theory study should not be. Many arguments abound in the literature and it is probably wise at this stage not to enter into that debate. These are complex arguments that you will find debated in the research methodology literature and while they should be acknowledged by the undergraduate researcher, they do not need to be addressed in any detail at this level. If you begin to engage with these arguments, you will enter a very complex area that will take you beyond what can be resolved at undergraduate level.

Three 'advanced' approaches for summing up the literature

Three of the well-known approaches for summing up the literature – meta-analysis, meta-ethnography and meta-study – are summarized below. It is important to note that these approaches offer a complex and comprehensive approach to the bringing together of results in a literature review and require the skills of experienced researchers. They are therefore generally beyond the remit of undergraduate study. It is, however, important that the novice researcher recognizes the terms that are used and can appreciate the rationale behind these approaches. Following their discussion, we look at a simplified approach to bringing together literature that has been adapted from the original approaches.

Meta-analysis

One approach for combining papers whose results are presented as statistics is meta-analysis. Meta-analysis was developed by Gene Glass in 1976 as a way of integrating and summarizing the statistical findings from a body of research. Glass described meta-analysis as 'the analysis of analyses', in which he refers to the 'statistical analysis of a large collection of results from individual studies for the purpose of integrating findings'. This process is referred to as meta-analysis and this approach was undertaken in the analysis described in Chapter 1, in which the results of the individual studies on the drug streptokinase were combined. Meta-analysis was used to combine the results of the studies and was able to demonstrate the effectiveness of the drug, a fact that was not apparent in the individual studies. The statistics from the different papers were combined to reduce the different sets of results to one bigger and more meaningful set of results. A meta-analysis of many different sets of results can only be undertaken if the studies included are similar to each other, so that the combination of results is meaningful. For example, if many randomized controlled trials (RCTs) concerning the same topic were identified, it would be possible to combine the results of these studies into one overall result. This has the advantage that the many and possibly varying results from each study are summarized into one study. However, unless the focus or design of all the studies is the same, combining the results will not be appropriate. It is important to note that meta-analysis refers to the statistical processes that are used to combine the results of the studies and that only studies of a similar nature can be combined. The limitations of using meta-analysis are that it is a complex process that may not be appropriate at undergraduate level. Furthermore, it is an approach that can be used only by those who have exclusively quantitative data of a similar type in their literature review.

Meta-ethnography

A commonly cited approach to the bringing together of qualitative research reports is meta-ethnography. This approach was developed by Noblit and Hare in 1988 and is regularly referred to by those reviewing qualitative data. Although the term 'meta-ethnography' seems to imply an ethnographic focus, in fact the method is applicable for all qualitative studies. Because it was devised specifically with ethnography in mind, the term was so named and although it is now a widely used approach across many qualitative methods, it has never been renamed. The authors describe their approach as the 'rigorous procedure for deriving substantive interpretations about any set of ethnographic or interpretive studies'

(Noblit and Hare 1988, p. 9). Meta-ethnography can be applied to all qualitative studies. The results of the qualitative studies are interpreted rather than summarized. Meta-ethnography involves determining keywords, phrases, metaphors and ideas that occur in all or some of the studies and to interpret these in the light of those identified in the other studies. The aim is to determine the relationship between the studies so that consistencies and differences are identified. New concepts are developed from the relationships identified. Meta-ethnography as defined by Noblit and Hare as a sophisticated approach to the combining of qualitative studies; however, the general principles can be applied to undergraduate study.

Meta-study

A third approach to the bringing together of qualitative research reports is **meta-study** as developed by Paterson *et al.* (2001). The authors offer an approach to the combination of studies that involves close examination of not only the data collected in each study, but also of the method by which the study is undertaken and the underlying theoretical framework upon which the study is based. Clearly, this approach demands a high level of expertise and research awareness training on the part of those who undertake it, and as such is generally beyond the remit of undergraduate study. However, as with meta-ethnography, the general principles can be adapted for use by the undergraduate student.

Limitations of these approaches for the novice researcher

The three established methods for bringing together papers identified for a literature review have been described. It will be evident from the discussion that there are limitations in the application of all these approaches at undergraduate level. First, none of the approaches can incorporate qualitative, quantitative and discussion papers with each other. Each approach is specific to either quantitative research (meta-analysis) or qualitative research (meta-ethnography or meta-study). Yet, there is growing recognition that literature from many different approaches may inform one research question and to leave out this literature because it is qualitative rather than quantitative (or vice versa) will not enhance the review. In health and social care, students are likely to encounter a wide variety of studies that are relevant to their research question rather than just one type of study. Second, all approaches require a high level of research expertise on the part of the researcher, beyond that which would be expected at undergraduate level.

Thematic analysis: a simplified approach

A thematic approach for summing up the literature that is suitable for those new to the literature review process will now be outlined. This method is simplified and adapted, the ideas for which have been generated from the work of those who have explored the analysis and synthesis of literature in further detail (Noblit and Hare 1988; Paterson *et al.* 2001; Walsh and Downe 2005; Bondas and Hall 2007; Finlayson and Dixon 2008; Rice 2008). This simplified approach has been used by many undergraduates to complete their literature reviews in health and social care and has been refined and amended according to the feedback and experience of those who have used it (Aveyard 2007, 2010).

Providing a critical summary of all your papers

The first step is to be able to summarize the content of all the papers and studies that you have. In the previous chapter, we discussed how it is important to undertake a critical appraisal of all the papers that you have and you may consider including these in the appendix of your dissertation. Whether or not these are included in your final thesis, the main point is that, as a result, you should have a detailed understanding of each of your papers, including the strengths and limitations of each. You will then be able to give an overall summary of the information you have found. As discussed in the previous chapter, you might find that one paper stands out as being particularly useful, owing to the detail that it gives, the strength of the critical appraisal or the method by which it was undertaken. You can use this 'core' or 'index' paper as a reference by which you judge the other literature that you have.

You might find it useful to compile a table to assist you in this process. An example is provided in Table 6.1.

The main purpose of this description is to give you an overview of all the studies you have, and the different approaches used in each one. It might be helpful to chart all the similar papers together within the chart. This will help you to clarify your understanding of the ways the papers relate to each other. You will also be able to keep track of the

Table 6.1 Summarizing your information

Author/date	Aim of study/ paper	Type of study/ information	Main findings/ conclusions	Strengths and limitations
Brown (2012)	To explore student views of campus life	Questionnaire study	35% of students preferred campus-based universities	Random sample of students not obtained. Very low response rate
George (2011)	To express opinion on campus life	Expert opinion	Campus-based universities prevent integration into the community	Anecdotal opinion only

authors of your papers so that you can reference them clearly when you write up your literature review.

Identifying themes

The second step is to begin to identify 'themes' from results of each study that you have. To start this process of identifying themes, go directly to the results section of each paper and re-read this section. If your paper is discussion only, then go to the general discussion section of the paper.

If you have predominantly research papers, then go through the main findings and consider how you might describe the findings the researchers present. You can use the terms used in the paper or you can paraphrase the findings in your own words. These descriptions will become the themes that you begin to identify. If you have mainly discussion papers or other reports, you can allocate themes to the main discussion points.

- Your themes are generated from the main findings or results of a paper; each research paper is likely to contain several themes that you can combine with the themes from other papers.
- The themes you generate should directly reflect the question you have set for your literature review.

When you allocate themes to the results of the different papers, try and think of words that summarize the main point that is made in that particular section. You might choose to annotate the paper using a highlighter pen to identify the themes. Go through all your papers undertaking this method until you have assigned a theme to all the results/discussion sections of the papers.

For example, let's say your literature review question relates to the childbirth experience of women with a physical disability. You have identified several papers that explore this and you commence the identification of themes. Each of these papers is qualitative. Below is an extract from the results of a paper by Tebbett and Kennedy (2012), the aim of which was to explore the childbirth experience of women who had a spinal cord injury. Suggested themes are presented in bold.

Example of the identification of a possible theme from the results of a research paper

Women discussed their anxieties regarding the uncertainty **anxiety**
about how their bodies would cope with the birth process **uncertainty**
and how aware of labour they would actually be.

(Tebbett and Kennedy 2012, p. 766)

As you read through the results of all the papers, you will identify more themes and you will begin to see how these themes fit together. It is useful to create a new table to tabulate the emerging themes and the papers they have been identified in. You will see that some of the themes arise in all papers and that some arise in only some of the papers. Tabulating these findings will help you to visualize the pattern of your results.

Developing your themes

Once you have allocated all the findings in the papers into themes, you need to merge all the data that have been allocated the same theme (Table 6.2).

There are different ways to manage this process:

- Some people 'cut and paste' the results from their papers into themes so that they capture the entire content of the results within each theme – do keep a second copy of the paper for reference if you use this approach. This can be a good way to proceed if you like to work visually.
- Others transcribe the theme onto an electronic document so that all the extracts about each theme are grouped together electronically – if you use this approach, remember to give as much detail and avoid summarizing the data so that you retain a full description.

Table 6.2 Developing your themes

Theme 1: Uncertainty	Theme 2: Anxiety	Theme 3: Role of partner	Theme 4: Coping strategies	Theme 5: Support gained
Tebbett and Kennedy (2012)	Tebbett and Kennedy (2012)	Another (2011)	Another (2011)	Another (2011)
Another (2009)	Another (2007)	Another (2006)	Another (2007)	Another (2009)
Another (2007)	Another (2009)	Another (2013)		Another (2007)
Another (2013)	Another (2006)	Another (2007)		Another (2013)

It is advisable to keep the original documents to hand at this point – do not put them to one side, as you will need to refer back to them to check for accuracy of the themes you are developing.

Discussion of the strength of evidence

You will probably consider giving more weight to research that provides stronger evidence than to weaker research. You will have identified this when you did your critical appraisal and even if you decided to include all papers irrespective of quality, you will find that you give more weight to the stronger papers in your final review. We will consider this further when writing up your review; at this point, you are probably aware which are the stronger studies and which are weaker, although you might change your opinion about this as your analysis develops.

Naming your themes

As you continue to develop your themes, you will need to consider a provisional name for the themes as they develop. It is important to emphasize that the names of the themes are provisional at this stage. As you continue to look at the results of the papers and your under-standing of the data develops, you may re-name your themes more appropriately.

Comparing the themes

The next step is to revisit each theme and check two things:

- Have you got the 'best fit' name for the theme?
- Do all the individual themes fit in the theme?

Lincoln and Guba (1985, p. 342) describe how this 'dynamic working back and forth' gives the researcher confidence that the development of themes is robust and open to scrutiny. Please note that Lincoln and Guba refer to themes as categories. You will need to check and re-check the accuracy of your theme development and expect to move data between the different themes until you get the 'best fit'.

Example

A theme might be labelled 'anxiety about hospital admission'. The data referred to within this theme that you identified from your literature might be 'patients' fear of hospital', 'distress at unfamiliar procedures', and so on. As you continue to develop your themes, you might feel that the data about 'distress at unfamiliar procedures' would better a theme on its own rather than be contained within the original theme.

This approach is similar to that carried out by qualitative researchers when they analyse qualitative data; for example, the methods outlined by Lincoln and Guba (1985). Paterson *et al.* (2001, p. 55) describe this process of coding and comparing studies in a literature review as a 'comparative analysis' of research findings. Through this process, the relationship of one study to another becomes apparent and there is continuous comparative analysis of the texts until a comprehensive understanding of the phenomena is reached (p. 64).

One of the main differences between the approach to meta-synthesis advocated in this book and the approaches developed by Noblit and Hare (1988) and Paterson *et al.* (2001) is the amount of detail that can be given to the analysis and synthesis of the results in each of the papers. For example, Paterson *et al.* (2001) recommend that two or three people code each paper to generate maximum insight about the meaning of the paper. At undergraduate level this is not likely to be possible, as resources do not permit; however, you might find it useful to discuss this process with your project supervisor or ask a friend or colleague to look over your ideas. If you do this, remember to write this up in your methods section.

Close scrutiny of your themes

It is at this point that the similarities and differences in the findings of your review will begin to emerge. Look closely at the themes you are developing and begin to consider how they are linked together. This is why it is important to keep the original documents near to hand, as you may need to refer back to them to check the information or to seek further information that becomes required as your analysis progresses. If you have 'cut and pasted' the results from the original papers and grouped these together into themes, you can refer back to the original sources easily. If you have compiled the themes electronically, make sure you refer back to the original sources so that you get the full meaning of the data. You will find that there are further questions you want to ask of the papers you have and will need easy access to them. For example, you might find that the experience of childbirth for women with a disability differs widely. However, on closer scrutiny, you identify that the age and marital status of the women seem to be linked to their experiences.

Working with themes that do not support each other

You might find that you have individual themes that do not support each other. The first thing to do is to consider the context of each paper from which the theme arose, together with the strengths and limitations of the research approaches undertaken. You need to return to your original critical appraisal of each paper at this point, as you need to re-assess the strength of the evidence in addressing your particular question. The rationale behind a review is that all the relevant literature is reviewed so that you can see each piece of literature in the context of the other available literature, and that differences and similarities in the results can be compared.

When you encounter literature that presents a different picture to that given by the previous literature you examined, it is important to document this carefully. Consider why this may be so. What were the differences in the pieces of research undertaken that may account for the different findings? Refer back to the critical appraisal you have undertaken. Is one piece of evidence stronger than the other? If no explanation is available, then you need to present the differing accounts and say that you cannot explain them. It is important to describe the differences in results that you find and not attempt to hide these in order to make your results appear to be more coherent. If all the data suggest different things, document this and say that you cannot reach firm conclusions from the data that you have.

For example, one small-scale study carried out on a small sample of participants might demonstrate different results from that obtained in a larger-scale study undertaken on a more representative sample. You would be more likely to give greater weight to the results of the larger study. The differences in the results might be explained by the sample sizes. Alternatively, one study set in an inner-city area might give very different results than a study undertaken in a rural area. Again, you would consider the relevance of these factors when considering the meaning of the results and you would consider which study setting is most applicable to your review.

You can also compare the results of research reports with non-research papers in this way, but again the contexts of both must be fully acknowledged. For example, a discussion paper by a leading expert might argue one point, but this point may not be borne out in the research studies that have addressed the same issues. You are likely to find research reports that contradict the opinion of an expert in the research topic area and vice versa. Consider again the widely opposing views of two leading environmentalists, David Bellamy and George Monbiot (Monbiot 2005). Again, when this is the case you need to consider which is the stronger evidence, expert opinion or a research study? Unless there are many identifiable flaws in the study, or you are specifically looking at expert opinion as part of your review, you are likely to conclude that the study provides the strongest evidence.

Be aware of results that appear too neat

It would be unusual if you were able to develop themes that presented an overall seamless picture in which there were no contradictory data. It is important to remember that there will always be inconsistencies that you cannot simply explain away. In such cases, you need to state that the findings of different studies do not appear to lead to the same conclusions and that it is beyond the scope of your review to explain this. Remember to include evidence of critical appraisal when you introduce each new paper that you include in your review.

Be creative!

The interesting part of this process is that the themes can be named as you deem appropriate. This is your analysis – be creative, but do be sure that you can justify the names of the themes and the relevant inclusion of data from the original studies. At the end of this process you should have a firmed-up set of themes with names that convey the meaning of the data within them.

Writing up your themes

When you write up your themes, it is important to remember that these themes are your findings and you should present them in a separate chapter. You should make this clear when you write up your review. They should be written up clearly in a section entitled 'themes or results or findings', just as you would find the results section in a piece of primary research. If you think back to the plan of a literature review, you can see how the presentation of the themes fits into the overall structure.

- a literature review question (or research question) set in context within an introductory chapter
- a methods section incorporating your search strategy, method of appraisal and analysis of the literature
- presentation of your results/themes incorporating critical appraisal of the studies included
- discussion of your results and recommendations for practice.

It is also important to remember that your themes should directly address the question you have set for your literature review. When you consider the titles of your themes, try to make sure that they address your literature review question so that you can demonstrate that you are using the themes to answer your literature review question.

Incorporating the results of the studies and critical appraisal in your themes

When you write up your themes, you need to incorporate the results of each paper contained within a particular theme and a concise critical appraisal of the study from which the data arose. Even if you include a detailed critical appraisal of each paper in an appendix, it is important to include reference to the critical appraisal process when you write up your themes. However, remember not to include a lot of detailed critical appraisal at the expense of describing the main findings in each theme!

The main component of each theme should be the findings/results from each of the research papers that are included within that theme. These should be described as fully and with as much detail as possible, as it is these findings that will help you to answer your question and enable you to compare one paper with another. In addition, you need to incorporate critical appraisal of the research into the description of your themes, so that you demonstrate that you are aware of the strengths of evidence that each paper brings to your literature review. As a general rule, at undergraduate level, you would expect to include a concise paragraph summarizing your critical appraisal of each paper you reviewed. This will be more extensive at postgraduate level. This paragraph should include the aims of the study, how it was conducted, and the strengths and weaknesses of the paper. You should include this the *first* time you refer to the paper in the first theme in which it appears. Subsequently, you do not need to include this critical appraisal summary each time you refer to this paper, but a short summarizing sentence is helpful, to remind the reader about the study mentioned previously.

- Remember to provide a reference for each paper reviewed within each theme. If you cite your references clearly within each theme, you will avoid any potential questions about the authority of the work.
- Remember to include a full description of the relevant findings from each research paper that contributes to your theme in addition to a concise paragraph of critical appraisal. The ratio of discussion of the findings to critical appraisal should be approximately 70:30 (findings 70 per cent; appraisal 30 per cent).

Examples of incorporating critical appraisal into your writing

---

Example 1 incorporates minimal critical appraisal
'Smith (2006) argues that nurses use their professional judgement when assessing wounds . . .' This sentence does not provide any reference to the context of the information from which this statement is drawn. There is no indication as to whether Smith is citing his or her opinion, someone else's opinion, or results from a study. You could argue that the statement is misleading.

Compare the above statement with the following example.

Example 2 incorporates more detailed critical appraisal

'Regarding the use of tools for the assessment of wounds, Smith (2006) explored how nurses assess the type of wound dressing they need for a particular patient. He interviewed ten experienced nurses working in a day care centre for older people in an urban hospital in England about their assessment strategies and how they applied these to different patients. He identified that while some nurses relied on the assessment tools available in the clinical area, many nurses relied on their clinical judgement. This was a small study, undertaken by a nurse experienced in the care of older people. All the interviews were tape-recorded and transcribed. However, all participants involved in the study were specialist practitioners with many years of experience. Those with less experience were not invited to participate in the study. The results are therefore not necessarily transferable to other settings.'

Example 2 contains more useful information than Example 1, yet both could be written with reference to the same study. This illustrates the need to provide a short critical appraisal of the literature you are using. When you then refer to this paper again, you need only to refer to the author and date of the paper.

Telling a story with your data

Once you have established your main themes, you need to present these in the most appropriate way to address your review question. You are likely to divide up your results section into a series of headings that relate to the main themes you have identified. You may begin the results section by describing the main finding or theme; that is, the theme that seems the most relevant to addressing your question or which contains themes that occurred most often in your literature. You should include all the research and other information that relates to this theme in this section. You will probably use research papers first followed by non-research papers. You are then likely to find that another theme illustrates an aspect of the first theme you present.

Again, you should include all the information relevant to this theme in this section. In this way, you will find that one follows on from another and gradually your research question is addressed in different ways by each of the themes you have identified. Your task is to organize these themes into a logical order so that the findings of one theme are then explained in more detail by the next, and so on. You also need to draw attention to themes that do not fit with the overall picture you are developing. Think of this process as being like telling a story – you are explaining how the literature you have identified addresses and sheds light on the research question you have selected.

What do I do if I cannot answer my literature review question?

Three scenarios are presented below that refer to the extent to which the literature addresses your research question. They are referred to as best-case, middle-case and worst-case scenario. They do not refer to the overall quality of your literature review but to the extent to which the available literature is able to answer the research question you identified.

The best-case scenario

The best-case scenario is where you have developed a set of categories, or themes, that relate to each other and fully address your research question. You are confident that each theme comprises information that is based on *strong evidence,* which is *at the top of your hierarchy of evidence,* and which is appropriate to answer your research question. You can then write these up, so that they tell a story and explain different aspects of the research question. Even with this best-case scenario, it is unlikely that all the aspects in each theme fit together – there will always be discrepancies and you will not always be able to explain these. However, you should document these inconsistencies.

The middle-case scenario

The middle-class scenario is where you have developed a set of categories or themes that relate in part to the research question or are comprised of evidence that is not very strong. You will need to comment on the strength of the evidence that makes up your theme and the relevance of this literature in addressing the research question. For example, one theme might address your question, but if the theme is composed of weak evidence, you need to address this and state that while there is some evidence that addresses your research question, the evidence is not strong and the results do not fully answer your question. You would be able to say that there is weak evidence to support a particular argument, but this cannot be further verified by the data that currently exists. In addition, you might be able to make theoretical arguments about the answer to your research question from the evidence provided. For example, if there is little available evidence on your research topic but there is evidence about a related topic, you might be able to theorize about the application of this knowledge to your topic. Remember that this evidence is not strong, but you might be able to make a good case. Remember also that not being able to answer a question is a useful finding in itself. You are now aware that the evidence does not exist to address your question. While this is not a comfortable finding, it is a useful finding.

The worst-case scenario

The worst-case scenario is that you find that none of your themes address your research question or that the evidence contained within the themes is very weak. For example, if your research question required empirical evidence such as results of primary data to address the question and you were not able to identify any studies involving primary data collection, you would have to conclude that the research question is not answerable. If this is the case, then you need to state that you have comprehensively and systematically undertaken all the steps required to review the literature in an attempt to address the (stated) research question but that the question was not answerable using the literature. This is an important finding in itself and points to the need for a study involving primary data collection in order to find an answer to the question you identified. At undergraduate level, you are less likely to be penalized for this; however, for those undertaking postgraduate study, you would be expected to have done a preliminary search of the literature to establish the viability of the research question before you commenced your study.

In reality, you will find that your evidence lies on a continuum where at one end your research question remains fully unresolved, while at the other your research question is completely addressed.

◄ - ►

Literature reviewed   Literature reviewed,
but does not address   completely answers
the research question   the research question

Tips for writing up your themes

1 You need to demonstrate how you developed the themes you describe.
2 Try to link the studies together so that you compare and contrast the studies.
3 Identify which studies/information do not fit into the overall argument you are making.
4 Identify any gaps in the literature that might leave aspects of your research question unanswered.
5 Remember to give a summary of your critical appraisal of each paper (when you write up your review) the *first* time you refer to it.

In summary

Throughout the process of summing up the literature, you are seeking to identify common themes that arise from the literature you have identified. You are likely to write up your themes under a series of main headings within which you discuss the main results within that theme. You are seeking to identify how the themes fit together, taking into account the strengths and limitations of the literature from which the themes are derived. Your task is then to organize your themes so that they relate to each other and follow a logical order. These themes should then be presented in a way that addresses the research question.

Key points

- Your main themes are the results of your literature review.
- The results of each paper included in your review should be scrutinized for themes that shed light on your literature review question.

- Ensure that you reference clearly each paper that you use.
- These themes are then brought together so that one theme expands on and adds insight to another.
- Remember to document where there are gaps in the literature that leave aspects of your question unaddressed.
- Remember to document information that does not fit with the argument you are making.

7

How do I discuss my findings and make recommendations?

- *Structuring your discussion*
- *Discussion of unanswered questions and future research*
- *Tips for writing up your discussion section*
- *Key points*

The final stage of your literature review is to bring your whole project together. This involves reflecting on the process you have undertaken and the way in which you can relate the main themes you have identified in your review to a wider context. This ultimately means that you have to interpret the meaning of your results and the implications they have on your area of practice. It is often reported that writing the discussion section of a dissertation or literature review is one of the hardest sections to write. Until this point, you have followed a systematic and logical process that has resulted in the presentation of the results of your study. How these results should be incorporated into the wider context can be a daunting task at the end of a study. If you are submitting your work for an academic degree, you might also be close to the deadline by which your work is to be submitted.

In order to do this, you need to look at your work critically, from different perspectives and with fresh eyes. If you can take a break from your review for a few days, you might consider your findings in a different light. Talk to others about your findings and their possible implications. Forget the detail for a moment, and consider the most important thing that your work has demonstrated – the aspects that you would most like to share with others. These are the aspects that you should bring out in your discussion.

Although it is important to emphasize that there is an interpretative element to your discussion, and even a creative side, it is also important to emphasize that your discussion must reflect the findings and themes you developed. Refer to your findings and themes specifically rather than making generalized statements such as 'all social workers do xx', if your data do not bear this out. Do not be tempted to exaggerate your findings so that your argument flows better. This will be identified by those who examine your work and your findings may be discredited. On the other hand, you do need to provide some interpretation of your findings and provide your own judgement of them. There is little point to a discussion section if you merely repeat the main findings of the study and do not exercise any judgement or interpretation of the findings (Skelton and Edwards 2000).

The most important thing to ensure is that the claims made in the discussion are actually borne out in the results. There is some general concern that some researchers interpret their findings too widely and make assertions that are not justified from the results obtained in the study (Doherty and Smith 1999). If your results are inconclusive, it is important to re-state this rather than try to make the results appear to show something that they do not. Be honest about what you have found; remember that finding little evidence about your literature review question is a useful finding in itself. It is better to be aware that an area needs researching than to assume that the practice we currently undertake is based on good evidence. Equally, if you have a lot of evidence about your literature review question, but the results are not what you expected or are equivocal, you must report this and be prepared to discuss the implications of an unexpected or inconclusive result.

Structuring your discussion

The following structure is a guide based on the work of Doherty and Smith (1999) and Drotar (2009) regarding how to present your discussion section. It is suggested that you follow this structure when writing up your discussion and attend to each of the following five points. Do note, however, that the section in which you discuss your findings should be the most substantial section in your discussion.

- Statements of findings
- Strength and limitations of your study
- Reflection of your role as researcher
- Discussion of your findings
- Recommendations and implications for practice.

Statement of findings

The first task is to summarize your findings. It is important to remember that you should not repeat the details of your results section in your discussion, but instead attempt to summarize your findings in one or two sentences that convey the general meaning of what your review has found. You are likely to require several attempts at the wording of this before you communicate succinctly the meaning of your findings. Try different ways, look objectively at the meaning of what you have written and consider whether you have captured the essence of your results in these sentences. It is appropriate to make generalizations about your findings when you are summarizing your results; for example, 'most social workers were happy to undertake additional duties however . . .', but you need to ensure that your generalizations convey the meaning of your findings. The important thing is that you capture the meaning of your results in a few sentences.

If you are able to summarize your findings in a few simple statements, this demonstrates that you have thought long and hard about what you have found in your review and have a good understanding of your findings. A lack of clarity about your findings often indicates a lack of clarity about your project as a whole.

Strengths and limitations of your study

It is important to acknowledge the strengths and limitations of your literature review. This is because it indicates to the reader the drawbacks to your research and enables the results to be placed in context. In the same way as you have undertaken a critical appraisal of the information upon which your literature review is based, it is also necessary to undertake a critical appraisal of your own work. Some possible limitations to your literature review might be as follows: as a novice researcher your approach to the identification, critique and bringing together of the literature may not have been as thorough as that of a more experienced researcher. In addition, there will have been time and resource limitations to your study. You are unlikely to have had the financial resources to commit to the study that might have enabled you to retrieve more literature via inter-library loans, or visiting libraries further afield. Additional finances might have enabled you to employ the assistance of other researchers who would have aided you in the search, critique and bringing together of the literature. Your study is also likely to have been limited due to time restraints. At this stage, you could also mention what you have learnt from undertaking this research process and how you would approach a similar study in the future.

Reflection of your role as researcher

It is also useful to comment on your developing role as a researcher. You might have never undertaken a literature review and you might consider a reflection on the journey you have taken, what you have learnt along the way and what you might do differently another time. You can be upfront about mistakes you made in the searching or critiquing process and comment on how you might approach this differently another time. You might also comment on whether you were surprised by the final outcomes of the review or whether they were in line with your expectations. Whereas you have attempted to retain a neutral stance throughout your dissertation, now is the time to show your true colours.

Discussion of your findings

This is the most important section of your discussion. The purpose of this section is to set your results within the wider context of your area of health and social care practice, research and theory.

If you are undertaking a literature review as a component of an academic degree, it is usually a requirement of the degree that the review relates specifically to the area of practice in which a qualification is sought. It is therefore important to explain the meaning of the results to your professional practice. If your degree is in management, then you need to emphasize the management focus of your findings. If your degree has a practical focus, then you need to emphasize this. Do not risk your degree by failing to achieve the required purpose of your dissertation.

There are two possible options to consider when discussing the findings of your review. The first is to discuss your findings *immediately after each theme*. In this way, the theme and the discussion are read consecutively so the reader can keep the flow of the argument. The alternative is to discuss your findings altogether *in a separate discussion section*. Whether you discuss your findings after each theme or in a separate section is up to you, but do inform your reader which approach you are taking. Whichever approach you take, remember to keep your results physically separate from your discussion so that everyone is aware of which papers you have used to address your research question and which are supporting papers. In some ways, these two options for discussing your findings reflect the two options often used by qualitative and quantitative researchers. It is common for qualitative researchers to discuss their results immediately after their findings, while quantitative researchers traditionally have a separate discussion section.

The main aims of your discussion of your themes is to begin to focus outwards and begin to consider how the main themes you have identified relate to the wider context in which your research question is located. This is where you begin to see the implications and relevance of your findings. Think widely about the area in which you are engaged in terms of government White Papers, consultation papers, professional guidelines, National Service Frameworks (if in the UK), and so on. You may have mentioned these in your introduction but you can refer back to them in your discussion in the light of the findings you have made. If you can refer your findings to policy or politics, then you can demonstrate the wider value of your work. Talk to experts in the area to check you have not missed any major developments that link into your topic area. Scan the 'news' sections of your professional journal, and continue to use the RSS feeds for debate that might add additional context to your review.

There are three main ways in which you can begin to compare your findings to a wider context: considering related research, policy or theory – or, indeed, a combination of these. To get started, consider the main themes that have arisen from your dissertation and start thinking a little more broadly. Consider whether you are most interested in comparing your themes with findings from other research, or with related policy or theory. If you are studying at postgraduate level, you are likely to be considering all three aspects in your discussion.

Relating your themes to further research

You might consider relating your themes to research in other related areas. For example, if your literature review focussed on a certain group of patients or clients, you could discuss your findings in the light of the findings of research that relate to a different group of patients or clients. For example, if your literature review question concerned the experiences of sports people in their rehabilitation following a knee injury, you might be interested in comparing your findings with the experience of sport people who have recently undergone rehabilitation following a shoulder injury. Or you might consider how the rehabilitation of athletes compares with that of a non-athletic population. Or if your literature review question concerned what it is like for homeless people to access medical or social care services, you might compare your findings with the experience of other 'hard to reach' groups. In this case, you will need to do some additional literature searches to identify papers that shed light on the topic of literature review question when it is related to other areas.

Relating your themes to relevant policy

You might consider relating your themes to local policy to see whether the findings of your review are in line with current policy. For example, if your literature review focussed on administration of medications and your results indicated that patients/clients prefer to administer their own medication while in hospital, you might compare how this finding fits in with local policy on the self-administration of medication. Alternatively, if your review found evidence that a particular professional role is highly valued by a particular patient/client group, you might explore how this role is perceived by those responsible for maintaining service provision.

Relating your themes to relevant theory

If you have related your literature review to a particular theoretical framework, now is the time to refer back to this and review your research in the light of this framework. For example, if your review focussed on what motivates people to lose weight, or to change any aspect of their behaviour, you can compare your findings with the current theory. A note of caution here, however though – unless you are undertaking a higher degree, you are unlikely to have the strength of evidence within a literature review to challenge established theory. But do feel free to comment with the proviso that you are aware of the limitations of your own review.

The extent to which you need to relate your findings to a wider source of existing evidence depends upon the level of degree award to which you are working. At undergraduate level, you do not usually need to undertake extensive further searches. It is more important to demonstrate that you can make links between the findings of your literature review and work in other but related areas. If you are working towards a higher degree, your discussion will be far broader.

Recommendations for practice

You should be able to identify some clear recommendations for practice. Remember that these arise from your own original work and so you can be bold about the assertions you make; however, you need to ensure that your recommendations arise directly from your discussion. It is useful to discuss these with your supervisor, as sometimes the recommendations can be subtle and can take a little teasing out. It is useful to give examples from your review to illustrate why the recommendations have been made. If your results are inconclusive, then you are likely to suggest that further research is needed. Recommendations can be listed clearly as bullet points.

Discussion of unanswered questions and future research

As has been discussed previously, it is very likely that when you undertake your literature review, you will not be able to answer your research question in full. You are likely only to be able to partially address the research question you have identified. This is because of the limitations in the data, or literature, you have collected. This may be due to *your* limitations as a researcher and the time restrictions you had, or it may be that there is little published information about your topic. It is therefore appropriate that you summarize what your research has failed to address and discuss the possibilities for future research. Depending on the strengths of the literature you have identified, further research might be either a further review of the literature or primary research for which your research has identified the need.

Tips for writing up your discussion section

1 Restate your research question when you commence this section.
2 Avoid repetition of the results section.
3 Do not add new ideas generated from your data to this section.
4 Be confident about the points you make. Remember this is your study and you are qualified to make assertions about practice and further research if they are justified.
5 You do not need to critique the research you refer to in the discussion but do demonstrate the link between your findings and related literature.
6 Finally, be clear as to how your findings have addressed the research question.

Key points

- Ensure your discussion is an accurate reflection of the results.
- Summarize your main findings in the discussion section, but briefly!
- Summarize the quality of the studies you included.
- Refer to related literature to set your study in context.
- Discuss any unanswered questions and recommendations for future research.

8

Frequently asked questions

- *How do I present my literature review?*
- *What is the difference between a dissertation and an essay?*
- *How should I structure my work?*
- *Should I use first or third person?*
- *How should I use references?*
- *How do I avoid plagiarism and misrepresentation?*
- *What is the role of my supervisor?*
- *Top tips for from the frequently asked questions*

How do I present my literature review?

Once you have undertaken all the work required to complete your literature review, you have one important task left. That is, to present your work in a way that reflects the hard graft that you have put in. The way in which your work is presented is very important. If you submit a carefully prepared report of your literature review, you will give the reader the impression that you have undertaken this piece of work in a careful manner. A hastily prepared report will give the opposite impression. It is also important that you follow a logical structure in the presentation of your work, so that the marker can see at a glance that you have been methodical in your approach to your study. Remember that if you do not write up any aspect of your literature review, the reader will assume that this aspect was not addressed in your work.

The following structure is suggested as a plan for your literature review. You are recommended to refer to the advice offered by your academic institution regarding the structure and layout of your literature review.

Title page and statement of authority

If you are submitting your literature review as part of an academic degree, you are advised to consult the guidance notes concerning the information required on your title page and whether you are required to complete a statement of authority.

Acknowledgements

It is customary to acknowledge your supervisor and any other professionals who have assisted your research in addition to others from whom you have received support.

Contents page

This should include appropriate reference to page numbers and include reference to appendices.

Lists of tables and figures

Include these, where appropriate, to illustrate your work.

Abstract

This is a very brief summary of the whole dissertation including the results and conclusions. Make sure it is an accurate summary of your research and findings.

Introduction

This usually explains your rationale for undertaking the study, provides an overview of the subject area and outlines your key research question(s). You will include background information in this section, defining key terms and referring to major research and/or theory that has been done or is relevant in the area. Remember that you do not have to include critical appraisal in this section, but it is useful to indicate whether the evidence you refer to is research or not. It is acceptable to summarize the main research in the area using key references.

Methodology and methods

This section incorporates every aspect of the systematic approach you have undertaken in order to achieve a comprehensive review of the literature. It is important that you document clearly how you undertook the steps involved. The reader needs to know that you followed a comprehensive and systematic approach to your literature review, and the only way to determine this is to give a full account of your literature review process. Do not leave this to chance. If you do not document a process that was undertaken, the reader will be given the impression that this process was not undertaken.

You might be asked to write both a methodology – an explanation and analysis of why you undertook a literature review – and a methods section – an explanation of the steps you took in undertaking your review. At undergraduate level it is often reasonable to combine these sections.

The methodology section will usually commence with how you identified your research question. Discuss the rationale for your research question and explore its origins. It is often useful to describe a critical incident that occurred in your practice that sparked your interest in the topic, if this is relevant. Then you need to address what was it about your research question that made it suitable for literature review rather than primary data collection.

In your methods section, you should then document how you searched for appropriate literature. You are advised to include a report of the search terms you used and your search strategy. Remember to document how many hits you had and how you identified relevant papers by comparing all the abstracts with your inclusion criteria. The research you identified as relevant to your review can be presented as in Table 6.1. You should then document how this literature was critiqued and justify your choice of critical appraisal tools. Finally, you need to document how you developed your themes and how you brought this information together. The process of generating themes can be documented as shown in Table 6.2. Overall, your methods section will contribute a large portion of the complete review and is likely to amount to approximately one-fifth to one-quarter of the total word count.

Results

This section incorporates the main themes/results that you have identified from the literature review. You are likely to commence with the most dominant theme and discuss the following themes thereafter. Remember to discuss all your themes in a logical order, bringing out the similarities and inconsistencies in the data that you have. Remember to give a short critical appraisal of each paper the first time you mention it in your results section.

Discussion

This section provides an interpretation of your results in the light of other related literature. It is important to ensure that your discussion draws on all aspects of your results section and that you do not add new information to your discussion section. In addition, you should set your results in context by exploring the limitations of your review. You should also discuss how your role as a novice researcher affected the ways in which the project was undertaken. Finally, you should discuss your role as researcher, how you have learnt from this role and what you would do differently next time.

References

There should be an exact match between the references you cite in the text and those in the reference list. You should reference every piece of published material to which you refer in your review. If you have used secondary references make sure you reference these as such. If your literature review is being submitted as part of an academic award, it is important to refer to the referencing guidelines issued by the academic institution to which you will be submitting it.

Appendices

These should contain any information that is relevant to your literature review but which is not contained in the main body of the text. For example, your completed critical appraisals of each paper and the processes by which you devised your themes when analysing the results of your literature search could be written up in the appendix. In addition, letters from practitioners or other professionals who assisted you in your research can be placed in the appendix. It is important to number each appendix.

What is the difference between a dissertation and an essay?

Students often ask about the differences between an extended essay and a dissertation. The difference between an essay and a dissertation is that in a dissertation you are seeking to develop professional knowledge. Up until the point of commencing your dissertation, the purpose of your essay writing has probably been for your own learning. You research a topic in some depth and write it up according to the instructions set by your academic institution. You are not seeking to develop knowledge or understanding in the area but rather to develop your own professional knowledge and promote your own learning. The aim of the dissertation process is not for your own learning, although it is clearly hoped that you will learn a lot along the way. Instead, the aim of the dissertation is to develop professional knowledge in the area you chose. For this reason, a dissertation always has a focussed research question that you seek to answer using an explicit method. The aim of this answer is to develop professional knowledge as you develop new insights from the literature you review.

For example, a dissertation question might be, '*What is the role of the social worker in supporting single parents of children under five years of age?*' The researcher might then explore the literature to determine what the prescribed roles are and how these roles are played out in practice. The review would be logical, systematic and organized, incorporating all the relevant research and policy concerning the role of the social worker. An essay on the same topic might be entitled '*What is the role of the social worker in supporting single parents?*' The essay writer would describe the main body of knowledge surrounding the role of the social worker in this context but would not follow the same systematic approach to the searching and management of the literature identified.

Broadly speaking, the differences between an essay and a dissertation are as follows:

- An essay is designed to promote your learning. A dissertation is designed to develop professional knowledge.
- If you are writing an essay, you are expected to summarize the main body of knowledge and information about a particular topic. If you are writing a dissertation, you are expected to develop a systematic approach to identifying and managing literature and to develop new

insights from the knowledge and information that has been written on the topic.
- The essay title is likely to have a broader scope than the dissertation research question.

While an exceptional essay might seek to develop new insights into a particular topic, a dissertation will always aim to do so. Additionally, a dissertation will have a clearly defined research question that is addressed by searching for, critiquing and reviewing the relevant literature in order to shed new light on the topic question.

Characteristics of an essay

- The focus of the topic can be broad.
- An essay will summarize current knowledge and information on a topic.
- The way in which knowledge is accessed is not necessarily made explicit.
- Textbooks may be referred to rather than original sources.

Characteristics of a dissertation

- The focus of the topic will be well defined and a research agenda will be set.
- A dissertation summarizes current knowledge prior to addressing the research question.
- A dissertation aims to identify all (or most) available evidence on a topic.
- Original sources are accessed and critically appraised.
- Analysis and synthesis of information is used to offer a new perspective on the topic and to answer the research question.

How should I structure my work?

The structure for a literature review should be coherent, systematic and clear (Hart 2003). This cannot be emphasized enough. It is very common, even for those who have used a systematic approach to the process of undertaking their dissertation, to find that this is not demonstrated through the writing up of their dissertation. One common occurrence is that the novice reviewer sets themselves a research question but then does not address the question. There can be a few reasons why this happens. First, the reviewer might not realize the importance of the research question. Second, the reviewer might encounter interesting information about a similar but not related topic and get sidetracked by this information. If this happens, you are advised, if circumstances permit, to alter your research question so that you can focus your research on a topic that has become more relevant to you. The worst thing you can do is to keep the research question unchanged but persevere with the literature that has caught your attention, if this does not relate to the question.

It is very important to keep your research question in mind throughout the whole process of undertaking your literature review. Some people find it useful to write the literature review question as a header on the entire document so that, at every stage of the writing, they can refer to their question. You also need to ensure that each chapter links into the previous chapter and then on to the next chapter. This can be achieved by providing a summary at the end of each chapter (a few sentences only) and then making specific reference as to how the next chapter takes the reader forward. For example, at the end of the first chapter, you might write something like: 'In this chapter I have argued why it is important to involve the social worker in the development of local policy for social housing. My research question seeks to address how this involvement can be achieved. In order to do this I intend to undertake a review of the literature. The methods I used to achieve this are outlined in the next chapter.'

Should I use first or third person?

Students often question whether they should write in the first or third person. That is, whether they should write 'I searched through CINAHL' or 'the author searched through CINAHL'. Some people feel that the third person form is more 'academic' and objective and therefore more appropriate for an academic piece of work. Other people feel that the first person assists clarity, especially when writing up the methods section and avoids any confusion as to which 'author' is being referred to; a literature review contains reference to many authors including the writer. On the other hand, use of first person can lead to an overly 'chatty' style whereas use of third person can seem overly 'formal'.

Unless you are required by your university to adopt either first or third person, the style in which you write is a matter of personal choice. The main thing is to aim for an academic style and clarity in your work. This is because when you are writing up your literature review, it is important that the process you undertook is explicit. You need to write in a way that reflects the experience you have had in undertaking the research process. In my view, the easiest way to achieve this is to write in the first person, so that it is clear who undertook the search, who undertook the critical appraisal, and so on. For example, 'I undertook an electronic literature search' is clearer than 'An electronic literature search was undertaken'. This is especially important when you are reviewing the literature because you are likely to be referring to many different authors and clarity is crucial. The passive voice can be useful in cases where you need to maintain anonymity, for example, 'I was informed that . . .' is preferable to 'XX informed me that . . .'. In summary, you need to ensure that your work is clear. If there is any uncertainty about who you are referring to when you state 'the author', you should use 'I' statements and restrict use of the term 'the author' for those whose work you are referring to.

How should I use references?

References should be used to provide evidence for the points you make throughout your literature review. In your introduction, methods and discussion sections you should use references to reinforce the points you make. Make sure you select a reference that illustrates the point you are making and that it is clear which aspect of your argument you are reinforcing with this reference. For example, if you are referring to the origins of evidence-based practice, you would be likely to refer to the work of Sackett *et al.* (1996). This is because their work was fundamental in establishing this approach to health and social care. If you cite a lesser known author who has discussed evidence-based practice and do not refer to the originators of the approach, you will not appear to have a comprehensive or thorough understanding of your topic. Therefore, it is important that you avoid the temptation to cite any reference that seems to reinforce the points you are making but that you trace the most relevant sources that reinforce your argument – even if the publication date is less recent. It can be useful to undertake a mini critical appraisal of the references you use so that you can be sure you are using the most appropriate ones. It is possible for those new to academic writing to perceive that any reference will enhance their written work as long as it relates in some way to the points they are making. In reality, if you cite an inappropriate reference, this will detract from the quality of your work. In principle, make sure the reference you cite is authoritative for the points you are making.

In your results section, you will use the references in far more detail. These references have been carefully identified from a thorough database search and additional searching strategies so you do not need to justify their inclusion. When you are writing up your themes, you are advised to give a short critical appraisal of each reference, the first time you cite this reference, so that the reader is aware of the type of reference you are using and can follow your arguments. If you refer back to this reference again in later themes, you do not need to repeat the critical appraisal. In this way, the reader can follow an audit trail of what literature is included in each theme and how you developed your themes.

How do I avoid plagiarism and misrepresentation?

Plagiarism refers to the presentation of the ideas and published material of someone else as if they were your own. This can be confusing for the novice researcher especially as the entire process of undertaking a literature review involves representing the work of others, analysing and summarizing this work in order to determine the contribution of this work in answering your research question. How you represent the work of others is clearly very important. There are a few general principles to follow:

1 When you refer to someone's work, always acknowledge the author, even if you are not making a direct quotation. The careful process of critical appraisal should lead you to be able to summarize the work of another researcher or practitioner in a way that does not lead to misrepresentation. It is important that you stay true to the literature that you have, so that you represent the information appropriately. Be sure to document all your references carefully as you go through the process of the literature review, so that all the sources you use are clearly referenced and your own ideas are identifiable from those of others.

2 Direct quotations of someone else's work must always be in quotation marks.
3 If you are referring to general ideas, you do not always need to provide a reference. However, if you do provide a reference, try to ensure that the reference is appropriate. For example, 'It is now well established that smoking causes cancer'. An appropriate reference should be made to the original studies that identified this link rather than any later commentary on the link between smoking and cancer. If you do refer to later commentaries on the link between smoking and cancer, you would need to discuss in which context you are using the reference.

What is the role of my supervisor?

If you are undertaking a literature review as part of an academic degree, you are likely to be allocated a supervisor. Your supervisor for your literature review is there as a resource, guide and support for your studies. He or she will not take the lead on the study and will expect you to determine the steps you need to take to complete your review. This is important at undergraduate level but essential at postgraduate level. When you meet your supervisor, be well prepared about the purpose of the meeting and what you need to achieve. You will waste valuable time if you are not prepared and do not use your supervisor time wisely.

Your supervisor might have a professional interest in your area of study, but this will not necessarily be the case. It is more important that your supervisor is familiar with the process of undertaking literature reviews than familiar with your topic area itself. This is because your supervisor will ensure that you are following the most appropriate ways to address your research question, rather than assisting you with the actual answer to that question. If your supervisor is not knowledgeable in your topic area, consider other ways in which you might find expert help that you can then feed back to your supervisor for further discussion. This will also help you to take the lead in the supervisory relationship.

When you begin the supervisory relationship, you are advised to discuss with your supervisor how you would like the supervision process to proceed. Discuss how you work, whether you respond well to deadlines or are sufficiently well motivated to set your own deadlines. Discuss when your supervisor would like to see drafts of your work and obtain information regarding the availability of your supervisor. Be clear regarding your expectations of your supervisor's role and where you should obtain extra support; for example, on information specifically related to your topic. Finally, consult carefully any guidance notes you may have on the role of the supervisor within your own institution.

Remember that your supervisor is unlikely to 'chase you up' regarding the process of your literature review. It is your project and you need to demonstrate that you are the project lead. Your supervisor is there to support you.

Top tips from the frequently asked questions

1   Ensure that you follow your research question throughout your review.
2   Every section that you write should relate to your question. If it does not, leave it out.
3   Make sure your review is coherent, systematic and clear.
4   Set your research question as the header or footer on your screen and adhere to it at all times.
5   Do not get sidetracked by unrelated issues and unrelated literature.
6   Keep a record of all references you use from the beginning of the literature review process.
7   Use either first or third person in your review.
8   Use references appropriately, as this will avoid any charge of plagiarism or misrepresentation.
9   Keep an up-to-date backup of your work.
10 Use your supervisor wisely.
11 Above all, make sure you answer the research question!

Glossary

Abstract: A summary of a research or discussion paper.

Action research: A study carried out in a setting in which the results are implemented and evaluated within that setting.

Analysing/analysis: The process of studying the relationship between different things; for example, the data collected for a research project or the results of different research projects.

Campbell Collaboration: a worldwide collaboration that commissions and maintains systematic reviews in social care.

Case control study: A study in which people with a specific condition (cases) are compared to people without this condition (controls) to compare the frequency of the occurrence of the exposure that might have caused the disease.

Clinical trial: a study undertaken in a clinical area to compare the effect of an intervention. The term clinical trial often refers to a randomized controlled trial.

Cochrane Collaboration: A worldwide collaboration that commissions and maintains systematic reviews in health care.

Cohort study: A study in which two or more groups, or cohorts, are followed up to examine whether exposures measured at the beginning lead to outcomes, such as disease.

Confidence interval: Confidence intervals are usually (but arbitrarily) 95 per cent confidence intervals. A reasonable, though strictly incorrect interpretation, is that the 95 per cent confidence interval gives the range in which the population effect lies.

CONSORT statement (Consolidated Standards of Reporting Trials statement): A statement that describes the information that should be included in the report of a trial.

Critical appraisal: A process by which the quality of evidence is assessed.

Critical appraisal tool: A checklist used to assess the quality of evidence.

Cross-sectional studies (surveys/questionnaires): Data that are gathered from a population at one point in time.

Database: A collection of data. In research, a database normally refers to a collection of journals that are searchable electronically.

Descriptive statistics: Statistics such as means, medians, standard deviations, which describe aspects of the data, such as central tendency (mean or median) or its dispersion (standard deviation).

Discussion papers: A paper presenting an argument or discussion; not a research paper.

Dissertation: A document presenting the main findings from a piece of academic work.

Empirical research: Research the opposite of empirical is theoretical. Empirical research is research that is based on observation or experiment.

Essay: A short piece of academic writing on a selected topic.

Ethnography: Qualitative research approach that involves the study of culture/way of life of participants.

Evidence-based practice (EBP): Practice that is based on the best available evidence, moderated by patient preferences.

Generalize: To apply the findings of a study to another population.

Grounded theory: Qualitative research approach that involves the generation of theory.

Hierarchy of evidence: A grading system for assessing the quality of evidence.

Hypothesis: A proposed explanation for an observable phenomenon.

Inclusion and exclusion criteria: Criteria that are set to focus the search strategy for a literature review (e.g. research from the past five years, published in English).

Information technology: The use of electronic computers to store, process and retrieve information.

Inferential statistics: Statistics that are used to infer findings from the sample population to the wider population, usually meaning statistical tests.

Keywords: Words that are central to the topic you are searching for, and used to search a database.

MeSH: Medical Subject Headings – a thesaurus of medical terms used to index medical information in some databases.

Meta-analysis: A process by which quantitative data with similar properties are combined to produce a weighted average of all the results.

Meta-ethnography: A process by which qualitative data are combined.

Meta-study: A process by which qualitative data are combined.

Meta-synthesis: A process of combining the statistical results of several studies that address a specific research question.

Mixed methods research: Research that incorporates two or more research methods in order to give different perspectives on a research question.

Narrative review: A literature review that is not undertaken according to a predefined and systematic approach.

Null hypothesis: An investigator proposes a study because he or she has a belief or hypothesis that one treatment is better than another. However, in statistical theory, it is not possible to prove a hypothesis. It is only possible to disprove one; therefore, the investigator sets up a hypothesis that they believe to be false (that there is no difference between the two treatments). This is called the null hypothesis. They then seek to falsify the null hypothesis: a hypothesis that proposes no relationship between the properties described in the hypothesis, for example, the null hypothesis that stated no relationship between lung cancer and smoking. This was disproved by research in the 1950s and 1960s.

Odds ratio: The odds of an event occurring in the experimental group, divided by the odds of an event occurring in the control group.

Phenomenology: Qualitative research approach in which the participants' 'lived experience' is explored.

PICOT: Acronym to assist literature review question formulation. The initials represent Population, Intervention/Issue, Comparison/Context, Outcome and Time – sometimes shortened to PICO.

Policy literature: Literature produced locally or nationally that publishes guidelines, policies and protocols.

Practice literature: Literature that describes what happens in practice.

Predefined question: A question that is set before the start of a research project or a literature review.

Primary research/research study: A study undertaken using a planned and methodological approach.

Purposive sampling: Sampling strategy used by qualitative researchers who are looking for a sample that is 'fit for the purposes' of the study in question.

P-values: P for probability. The P-value is the probability of observing results or results more extreme than those observed if the null hypothesis was true.

Qualitative data: Data that are collected for a qualitative study.

Qualitative research: Research that involves an in-depth understanding of the reasons for and meanings of human behaviour.

Quantitative research: Research that involves counting.

Questionnaire: A list of questions to be asked of respondents.

Random sampling: A sampling strategy in which everyone in a given population has an equal chance of being selected and that probability is independent of any other person selected.

Randomization/random allocation: The process of allocating individuals randomly to groups in a trial.

Randomized controlled trial (RCT): A trial that has randomly assigned groups in order to determine the effectiveness of an intervention(s) that is given to one/two of the groups.

Research literature: Literature that describes and reports a research project or study.

Research methodology: The process undertaken to address the research question.

Research question: A question set by researchers at the outset of a study, to be addressed in the study.

Research study/primary study: A study undertaken using a planned and methodological approach.

Rigour: evidence that the research has been carried out in a robust manner.

Risk ratio: The ratio of risk of an event occurring in the experimental group divided by the risk in the control group

Sample: The group of people included in a study

Search strategy: A predefined plan for searching for information or research on a topic.

Secondary source: A source that is not derived from an eyewitness account of a situation.

Snowball sampling: A sampling strategy in which who/what is involved in the study (sample) is determined according to the needs of the study as the investigation progresses.

SPIDER: Acronym to assist literature review question formulation. The initials represent Sample, Phenomena of Interest, Design, Evaluation, Research.

Statistics: Descriptive and inferential statistics (defined above).

Stratification: Stratification is when the sample is divided into groups that have the same value; for example, stratifying by age means putting people of the same age or age group together.

Strict protocol: A predefined method for undertaking a research project or literature review.

Subject-specific electronic databases: Databases containing collections of journals relevant to a specific professional topic.

Systematic review: A review of the literature that is undertaken according to a defined and systematic approach.

Theoretical framework: A background of theoretical literature that helps to set the findings of a study or literature review in context.

Theoretical literature: Literature that describes a theory or a set of ideas.

Theoretical sampling: An approach to sampling in grounded theory where the sampling strategy evolves as the study progresses, according to the needs of the study and the developing theory.

Transferability: The results of a study may be transferred to another context or population.

Validity: The extent to which a study or an intervention measures what it is intended to measure.

References

Anderson J, Malley K and Snell R (2009) Is 6 months still the best for exclusive breastfeeding and introduction of solids? A literature review with consideration to the risk of the development of allergies, *Breastfeeding Review* 17(2): 23–31.

Arksey H and O'Malley K (2005) Scoping studies; towards a methodological framework, *International Journal of Social Research Methodology* 8(1): 19–32.

Aveyard H (2007) *Doing a Literature Review in Health and Social Care*. Maidenhead: Open University Press.

Aveyard H (2010) *Doing a Literature Review in Health and Social Care* (2nd edn.). Maidenhead: Open University Press.

Aveyard H and Sharp P (2013) *A Beginner's Guide to Evidence Based Practice* (2nd edn.). Maidenhead: Open University Press.

Aveyard H, Sharp P and Woolliams M (2011) *A Beginner's Guide to Critical Thinking and Writing*. Maidenhead: Open University Press.

Barbour RS (2001) Checklists for improving rigour in qualitative research: a case of the tail wagging the dog?, *British Medical Journal* 322: 1115–17.

Barnett-Page E and Thomas J (2009) Methods for the synthesis of qualitative research: a critical review, *BMC Medical Research Methodology* 9: 59.

Beed B (2012) *The experience of nurses caring for potential and actual organ donors in intensive care*. Unpublished BSc dissertation, Oxford Brookes University, Oxford.

Betrán AP, Say L, Gülmezoglu AM, Allen T and Hampson L (2005) Effectiveness of different databases in identifying studies for systematic reviews: experience from the WHO systematic review of maternal morbidity and mortality, *BMC Medical Research Methodology* 5: 6.

Bondas T and Hall EOC (2007) Challenges in approaching metasynthesis research, *Qualitative Health Research* 17: 113–21.

Bradshaw A (2001) *The Nurse Apprentice 1860–1977*. Farnham: Ashgate Publishing.

Caroll C, Booth A and Lloyd Jones M (2010) *Should we exclude poorly conducted qualitative studies from systematic reviews? An evaluation of reviews of qualitative data*. Oral presentation at the joint Cochrane/Campbell Colloquium, Keystone, CO, 18–22 October.

Childs A (2012) *What does evidence show are the most effective treatment/support options for homeless adults with a dual diagnosis of mental health and substance use issues?* Unpublished MSc dissertation, Oxford Brookes University, Oxford.

Cooke A, Smith D and Booth A (2012) Beyond PICO: the SPIDER Tool for qualitative evidence synthesis, *Qualitative Health Research* 22(10): 1435–43.

Cottrell S (2005) *Critical Thinking Skills*. Basingstoke: Palgrave Macmillan.

Crombie I (2006) *Pocket Guide to Critical Appraisal*. London: BMJ Publishing Group.

Crowe M and Sheppard I (2011) A review of critical appraisal tools show they lack rigor: alternative tool structure is proposed, *Journal of Clinical Epidemiology* 64(1): 79–89.

Department of Health (2012) *Smoking Health Harm Campaign*. Available at: http://www.dh.gov.uk/health/2012/12/smoking-health-harm/.

Dixon-Woods M, Sutton A, Shaw R, Miller T, Smith J, Young B *et al.* (2007) Appraising qualitative research for inclusion in systematic reviews: a quantitative and qualitative comparison of three methods, *Journal of Health Service Research Policy* 12(1): 42–7.

Doherty M and Smith R (1999) The case for structuring the discussion of scientific papers, *British Medical Journal* 318: 1224–5.

Doll R and Hill AB (1954) The mortality of doctors in relation to their smoking habits, *British Medical Journal* 1: 1451–5.

Drotar D (2009) Editorial: How to write an effective results and discussion for the Journal of Pediatric Psychology, *Journal of Pediatric Psychology* 34(4): 330–43.

Evans D (2003) Hierarchy of evidence: a framework for ranking evidence evaluating health care interventions, *Journal of Clinical Nursing* 12: 77–84.

Faden R and Beauchamp T (1986) *A History and Theory of Informed Consent*. New York: Oxford University Press.

Faggiano F, Vigna-Taglianti FD, Versino E, Zambon A, Borraccino A and Lemma P (2006) School based prevention for illicit drug use, *Cochrane Database of Systematic Reviews* 2: CD003020.

Fineout-Overholt E and Johnston L (2005) Teaching evidence based practice: asking searchable, answerable clinical questions, *World Views on Evidence-based Nursing* 2(3): 157–60.

Finfgeld DL (2003) Metasynthesis: the state of the art so far, *Qualitative Health Research* 13(7): 893–904.

Fink A (2005) *Conducting Research Literature Reviews*. Thousand Oaks, CA: Sage.

Finlayson KW and Dixon A (2008) Qualitative meta-synthesis: a guide for the novice, *Nurse Researcher* 15(2): 59–71.

Florence Z, Schulz T and Pearson A (2005) *Inter-reviewer agreement: an analysis of the degree to which agreement occurs when using tools for the appraisal, extraction and meta-synthesis of qualitative research findings*, Presentation at the XIII Cochrane Colloquium, 22–26 October, Melbourne, VIC, Australia.

Giustini D (2005) How Google is changing medicine, *British Medical Journal* 331: 1487–8.

Glaser BG and Strauss A (1967) *The Constant Comparative Method of Qualitative Analysis: The Discovery of Grounded Theory*. Chicago, IL: Aldine.

Glass GV (ed.) (1976) *Evaluation Studies Review Annual*, Vol. 1. Beverly Hills, CA: Sage.

Goldacre B (2012) *Bad Pharma: How Drug Companies Mislead Doctors and Harm Patients.* London: Fourth Estate.

Greenhalgh T (1997) How to read a paper: papers that summarise other papers, *British Medical Journal* 315: 672–5.

Greenhalgh T (2010) *How to Read a Paper: The Basics of Evidence Based Practice.* London: Wiley-Blackwell/BMJ Books.

Greenhalgh T and Peacock R (2005) Effectiveness and efficiency of search methods in systematic reviews of complex evidence: audit of primary sources, *British Medical Journal* 331: 1064–5.

Guba EG and Lincoln YS (1995) *Fourth Generation Evaluation.* Newbury Park, CA: Sage.

Hannes K and Lockwood C (2011) Pragmatism as the philosophical foundation for the Joanna Briggs meta-aggregative approach to qualitative evidence synthesis, *Journal of Advanced Nursing* 67(7): 1632–42.

Harden A (2007) *Does study quality matter in systematic reviews which include qualitative research?*, Oral presentation at the XV Cochrane Collaboration Colloquium, 23–27 October, Sao Paulo, Brazil.

Hart C (2003) *Doing a Literature Review.* London: Sage.

Hek G, Langton H and Blunden G (2000) Systematically searching and reviewing literature, *Nurse Researcher* 7(3): 40–58.

Horsburgh D (2003) Evaluation of qualitative research, *Journal of Clinical Nursing* 12: 307–12.

Jensen LA and Allen MN (1996) Meta-synthesis of qualitative findings, *Qualitative Health Research* 6(4): 553–60.

Katrak P, Bialocerkowski AE, Massy-Westropp N, Kumar S and Grimmer KA (2004) A systematic review of the content of critical appraisal tools, *BMC Medical Research Methodology* 4(22): 22–33.

Kmietowicz Z (2012) University College London issues new research standards but says it won't investigate Wakefield, *British Medical Journal* 345: e6220.

Knipschild P (1994) Systematic reviews: some examples, *British Medical Journal* 309: 719–21.

Kvale S (1989) *Issues of Validity in Qualitative Research.* Thousand Oaks, CA: Sage.

Law R (2004) From research topic to research question: a challenging process, *Nurse Researcher* 11(4): 54–66.

Light RJ and Pillemer DB (1984) *Summing Up: The Science of Reviewing Research.* Cambridge, MA: Harvard University Press.

Lincoln YS and Guba EG (1985) *Naturalistic Inquiry.* Beverly Hills, CA: Sage.

McKibbon KA, Wilczynski NL and Haynes RB (2006) Developing optimal search strategies for retrieving qualitative studies in PsycINFO, *Evaluations and the Health Professions* 29(4): 440–54.

Mattioli S, Farioli A, Cooke RM, Baldasseroni A, Ruotsalainen J, Placidi D *et al.* (2012) Hidden effectiveness? Results of hand-searching Italian language journals for occupational health interventions, *Occupational and Environmental Medicine* 69(7): 522–4.

Moher D, Liberati A, Tetzlaff J, Altman DG and The PRISMA Group (2009) *Preferred Reporting Items for Systematic Reviews and Meta-Analyses*: The PRISMA Statement, *Annals of Internal Medicine* 151(4): 264–9.

Monbiot G (2005) Junk science, *The Guardian*, 10 May.

Morse JM (1994) 'Emerging from the data': the cognitive processes of analysis in qualitative inquiry, in *Critical Issues in Qualitative Research Methods*. London: Sage.

Morse JM (1999) Qualitative generalisability, *Qualitative Health Research* 9(1): 5–6.

Morse JM, Barrett M, Mayan M, Olson K and Spiers J (2002) Verification strategies for establishing reliability and validity: qualitative research, *International Journal of Qualitative Studies* 1(2): 1–19.

Mulrow CD (1994) Systemic reviews: rationale for systematic reviews, *British Medical Journal* 309: 597–9.

Mulrow CD, Cook DJ and Davidoff F (1997) Systematic reviews: critical links in the great chain of evidence, *Annals of Internal Medicine* 126(5): 389–91.

Noblit GW and Hare RD (1988) *Meta-ethnography: Synthesizing Qualitative Studies*. Qualitative Research Methods Series, Vol. 11. London: Sage.

Noyes J and Popay J (2007) Directly observed therapy and tuberculosis: how can a systematic review of qualitative research contribute to improving services? A qualitative metasynthesis, *Journal of Advanced Nursing* 57(3): 227–43.

O'Connor D, Green S and Higgins JPT (2008) Defining the review question and developing criteria for including studies, in JPT Higgins and S Green (eds.), *Cochrane Handbook for Systematic Reviews of Interventions*. Chichester: Wiley.

Offit P (2013) *Killing Us Softly: The Sense and Nonsense of Alternative Medicine*. London: Fourth Estate.

Oppenheim AN (1992) *Questionnaire Design, Interviewing and Attitude Measurement*. London: Continuum.

Papaioannou D, Sutton A, Carroll C, Wong R and Booth A (2010) Literature searching for social science systematic reviews: consideration of a range of search techniques. *Health Information and Libraries Journal* 27(2): 114–22.

Paterson B, Thorne S, Canam C and Jillings C (2001) *Metastudy of Qualitative Health Research*. Thousand Oaks, CA: Sage.

Pauling L (1986) *How to Live Longer and Feel Better*. Corvallis, OR: Oregon State University Press.

Pirie K, Peto R, Reeves GK, Green J and Beral V (2013) The 21st century hazards of smoking and benefits of stopping: a prospective study of one million women in the UK, *The Lancet* 381(9861): 133–41.

Pleasance ED, Stephens PJ, O'Meara S, McBride DJ, Meynert A, Jones D *et al.* (2010) A small cell lung cancer genome reports complex tobacco exposure signatures, *Nature* 463(7278): 184–90.

Polit DF and Beck C (2010) *Essentials of Nursing Research* (7th edn.). Baltimore, MD: Lippincott Williams & Wilkins.

Popay J, Rogers A and Williams G (1998) Rationale and standards for the systematic review of qualitative literature in health services research, *Qualitative Health Research* 8(3): 341–51.

Prochaska JO, Norcross JC and DiClemente CC (1994) *Changing for Good.* New York: William Morrow.

Rice MJ (2008) Evidence-based practice in psychiatric and mental health nursing: qualitative meta-synthesis, *Journal of the American Psychiatric Nurses Association* 14(5): 382–5.

Rochon PA, Gurwitz JH, Sykora K, Mamdani M, Streiner DL, Garfinkel S *et al.* (2005) Reader's guide to critical appraisal of cohort studies: 1. Role and design, *British Medical Journal* 330: 895–7.

Russell CK and Gregory DM (2003) Evaluation of qualitative research studies, *Evidence Based Nursing* 6: 36–40.

Sackett DL, Rosenberg WMC, Muir Gray JA, Haynes RB and Richardson WS (1996) Evidence based medicine: what it is and what it isn't, *British Medical Journal* 312: 71–2.

Sandelowski M and Barroso J (2002) Reading qualitative studies, *International Journal of Qualitative Studies* 1(1): 1–47.

Sandelowski M, Docherty S and Emden C (1997) Qualitative metasynthesis: issues and techniques, *Research in Nursing and Health* 20: 365–71.

Schulz KF, Altman DG and Moher D (2010) CONSORT 2010 Statement: updated guidelines for reporting parallel group randomised trials, *British Medical Journal* 340: 332.

Shin KR, Kim MY and Chung SE (2009) Methods and strategies utilized in published qualitative research, *Qualitative Health Research* 19(6): 850–8.

Skelton J and Edwards SLJ (2000) The function of the discussion section in academic medical writing, *British Medical Journal* 320: 1269–70.

Tang H and Ng JHK (2006) Googling for a diagnosis – use of Google as a diagnostic aid: Internet based study, *British Medical Journal* 333: 1143–5.

Tebbett M and Kennedy P (2012) The experience of childbirth for women with spinal cord injuries: an interpretative phenomenological analysis study, *Disability and Rehabilitation*, 34(9): 762–9.

Thomas J and Harden A (2008) Methods for the thematic synthesis of qualitative research in systematic reviews, *BMC Medical Research Methodology* 8: 45.

Thorne SE (2001) The implications of disciplinary agenda on quality criteria for qualitative research, in J Morse, JM Swanson and AJ Kuzel (eds.) *The Nature of Qualitative Evidence.* Thousand Oaks, CA: Sage.

Thouless RH and Thouless CR (1953) *Straight and Crooked Thinking* (4th edn.). London: Hodder & Stoughton.

Tong A, Sainsbury P, Craig J (2007) Consolidated criteria for reporting qualitative research (COREQ): a 32 item checklist for interviews and focus groups. *International Journal for Quality in Health Care* 19(6): 349–57.

Wakefield AJ, Murch SH, Anthony A, Linnell J (1998) Ileal-lymphoid-nodular hyperplasia, non-specific colitis and pervasive developmental disorder in children, *The Lancet* 351: 637–41 (paper now withdrawn).

Walker S (2013) Undiagnosed breech birth: towards a woman centered approach, *British Journal of Midwifery* 21(5): 316–22.

Wallace M and Wray A (2006) *Critical Reading and Writing for Postgraduates.* London: Sage.

Walsh D and Downe S (2005) Meta-synthesis method for qualitative research: a literature review, *Journal of Advanced Nursing* 50(2): 204–11.

Wellcome Trust (2010) One mutation per 15 cigarettes: genome maps reveal how cancer develops. Available at: http://www.wellcome.ac.uk/News/2010/News/WTX058965.htm.

West R (2006) *Theory of Addiction.* Oxford: Addiction Press/Blackwell Publishing.

Whitlock EP, Lin JS, Chou R, Shekelle P and Robinson KA (2008) Using existing systematic reviews in complex systematic reviews, *Annals of Internal Medicine* 148: 776–82.

Wilczynski NL, Marks S and Haynes RB (2007) Search strategies for identifying qualitative studies in CINAHL, *Qualitative Health Research* 17(5): 705–10.

Wise J (2013) Largest group of children affected by measles outbreak in Wales are 10–15 year olds, *British Medical Journal* 346: f2545.

Wong SS, Wilczynski NL, Haynes RB and the Hedges Team (2004) Developing optimal search strategies for detecting clinically relevant qualitative studies in MEDLINE, *Medinfo: Studies in Health Technology and Information* 107(1): 311–16.

Woolliams M, Williams K, Butcher D and Pye J (2009) *Be More Critical! A Practical Guide for Health and Social Care Students.* Oxford: Oxford Brookes University.

Index